THIS BOOK MAY
SAVE YOUR LIFE

THIS BOOK MAY
SAVE YOUR LIFE

DR KARAN RAJAN

1 3 5 7 9 10 8 6 4 2

Century
20 Vauxhall Bridge Road
London SW1V 2SA

Century is part of the Penguin Random House group of companies
whose addresses can be found at global.penguinrandomhouse.com

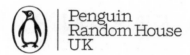

First published by Century in 2023

www.penguin.co.uk

A CIP catalogue record for this book is available from the British Library.

ISBN 9781529136326

Typeset in 9.75/13.5pt Gill Sans MT Pro by Jouve (UK), Milton Keynes
Printed and bound in Great Britain by Clays Ltd, Elcograf S.p.A.

The authorised representative in the EEA is Penguin Random House Ireland,
Morrison Chambers, 32 Nassau Street, Dublin D02 YH68

www.greenpenguin.co.uk

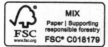

MIX
Paper | Supporting
responsible forestry
FSC® C018179
www.fsc.org

Penguin Random House is committed to a
sustainable future for our business, our readers
and our planet. This book is made from Forest
Stewardship Council® certified paper.

CONTENTS

INTRODUCTION

LET ME DESCRIBE MY JOB in non-medical terms. I slice into people when they're asleep (with their consent) and remove things. I should stress that I'm one of the good guys, because despite missing some stuff from their bodies, when they surface my patients feel more whole as a result. As a general surgeon, I have the pleasure of dealing with everything from guts to gall bladders, bleeding haemorrhoids and beyond.

Over the course of my career, I've had the blessing and misfortune to witness everything from miracle surgeries to tragic losses. In the process, I've come to appreciate that the human body is both a miracle of biology and a total deathtrap.

This book is not a medical encyclopedia. Nor will it qualify you as a doctor. You can pretty much pick up all the medical skills you need on Google nowadays. At least that's what some people are led to believe. Instead, what's on offer here is the extraordinary story of how your incredible body is also out to destroy you.

It's not all doom and gloom. Having witnessed my rose-tinted view of the human body darken from the moment I entered medical school, and continue to dim through all my years of unpicking problems, faults and breakdowns inside my patients, I thought it would be useful to create a survival guide to this meat suit in which you're trapped for life. If you're familiar with my work on TikTok – where I started out posting about how to perform the perfect poo and found the brand of milkshake that drew millions of people to my yard – you'll know that I enjoy busting body myths and exploring subjects that should never have become taboo. When it comes to health, <u>not</u> talking about personal issues does us humans a massive disservice. So, let's right that wrong here in one book, which you can read for entertainment, education, or as a hacker's guide to getting the most out of your body.

Ultimately, I'm here to guide you safely around your body's biological barbs, traps, slides and pitfalls to improve your quality of life. Maybe you'll fine-tune your sleep health, say goodbye to indigestion or simply enjoy the most epic and efficient dump of your existence. At the very least it might help to slow the inevitable decay your body started going through from the moment of your birth. Ultimately, my sincerest hope is that this book serves as an instruction manual to our eventual AI overlords, so they know how to take care of a human and get the most out of us.

I first crossed paths with medicine in 1996. On a particularly humid afternoon in the suburbs of Mumbai, I was playing a game of street cricket with my cousin. As he ran up to bowl towards me, he was struck by an invisible force and crumpled to the ground in agony. It was a terrifying moment. I felt so helpless, and that helplessness had a profound effect on me. Having helped my family rush him to hospital, we spoke to the doctors who diagnosed him with a ruptured appendix. I didn't really know what that meant at the time but seeing him drop down opened my eyes to a simple truth: the human body is awesome, but seems hell-bent on taking us out.

At medical school interviews, where I found myself after having decided upon my calling, they always love to dredge up the same question: 'Why do you want to do medicine?' Predictably, everyone churns out the same panicky, unimaginative drivel which broadly revolves around two main themes. Firstly, 'I want to help people' and secondly, 'I'm fascinated by the human body . . .'

Anyone who truly knows me (which, due to my long and antisocial shift hours, is kind of limited to my parents) could have told you that the first reason never really applied to me. I like people, and if I can save their lives I'm thrilled, but ultimately, I am driven by an obsession with how the body works. It's only now, however, when I look back at my career, that I realise that it's not the kind of wide-eyed fascination which we tend to express watching wildlife documentaries fronted by Sir David Attenborough. The truth is I'm a little bit like a bystander at a traffic accident. I can't stop looking, despite my better nature, because I am appalled at what I'm witnessing. Having lost count of the number of surgical operations I've conducted, and become hands-on familiar with the body's inner workings, I can confidently say that it's a miracle that we're even here as a species.

You're basically a living, breathing canvas of hand-me-down traits, and that includes structures that seemingly serve no purpose. Take chins, for example. Even our close cousins Homo erectus and the Neanderthals didn't feel the need to sport them. Ultimately, you just have to be content with the fact that you're the sum total of a lot of mistakes, trials and errors. It's just that evolution has buried the evidence. Mostly.

Throughout my time in medical school, I loved to get under the skin. Above all, I was drawn to the practical anatomy sessions. I dissected into abdominal muscles and uncovered the full length of the intestines, various blood vessels and a network of nerves that ran through the body like phone lines. This behind-the-scenes view of life felt invasive and unnatural but also essential. It was here that I decided I was going to become a surgeon. It would be an opportunity to understand how our bodies are equipped to wipe us out, but also how we can enhance them, or tweak our lifestyles, to minimise the chances of falling apart before our time is due.

We focus so much of our everyday lives on the external appearances of things and often relegate our internal organs to the recesses of our mind. The body is a family and each member – from the liver and stomach to the heart and brain – has their specific part to play in keeping us alive. Just like any family, however, everyone relies on each other for support. So, when one goes rogue, or members fall out with each other, the whole family can implode.

I fell in love with this occasionally dysfunctional family over the course of six years at medical school. Throughout this time, I spent countless hours staring at cellular architecture under a microscope, dissecting dead bodies in cadaver labs and meeting patients who taught me how the body performs in both sickness and health. Finally, I traded in the lecture slides and multiple-choice questions and started hospital rotations.

My first was general surgery.

The night before I started, I rigorously revised my gastrointestinal anatomy. If I was to be grilled by the surgeons on the minutiae of the blood supply to the large intestine, I refused to find myself afflicted by the dreaded condition I'd heard about called hotseat aphasia (aphasia is the inability to speak, often affecting patients who've had strokes but can also transiently affect nervous medical students when they are under the spotlight).

I was scrubbed into an operation to remove a bowel cancer, but it all seemed so vastly different from the textbooks. I was also far removed from the serene environment of the cadaver lab, where you could explore organs at a gentle pace and prod and poke with curiosity. When the surgeon made the cut into the abdominal tissue, a small jet of red fluid hit my nose. This was real medicine. A living human being had placed their life in our hands.

The incision that the surgeon opened up revealed a glistening, moist interior, like wet velvet. With the patient's chest rising and falling, I peered into the abdominal cavity to see the intestines, bathed in a straw-coloured juice, wriggling like a bowl of worms. At that point the anaesthetist alerted us to the fact that the bleeding had caused the patient's heart rate to go up and the blood pressure to drop. The trauma we had introduced with that scalpel had caused their breathing to become laboured. Such observations finally revealed to me that my learnings so far had been flawed. It was only now that I realised how distant organs, seemingly disconnected, were like tenants living in a shared flat. If one person clogs the toilet, everyone is affected.

Showing the kind of calm under pressure that took me a while to acquire, the surgeon worked quickly and skilfully to complete the procedure. With the patient stabilised, and the tumour removed, it struck me that the experience had been life-changing for more than one of us.

Medicine is an industry for specialists. Doctors have become increasingly narrowed in their scope of expertise, veering away from their predecessors who maintained a basic grasp of every field. This is a good thing, especially if you're the one being treated, because ultimately you want to feel confident that the surgeon removing your gall bladder is a master of the procedure and hasn't just memorised a YouTube tutorial. Even though I mainly deal with guts these days, I find it still helps for me to see the human body as a whole. After all, one variable can cause the entire system to alter and even falter. This balance, sometimes referred to as homeostasis, is crucial for optimal human function. I'd like to reassure you that the major players inside your body have mastered their interconnected requirements with the kind of orchestral choreography that invites praise and applause from every seat in the theatre. It's just having witnessed the chaos behind the scenes, I can't join in with the clapping.

So, while I will be the first to celebrate the marvels of the human body in the journey you're about to undertake, I won't hold back on the flaws, shonky designs and cack-handed wiring that make it so unique. For all its faults, however, this organic life support system that you're on provides ample opportunity for customisation and even improvement. It's just a question of understanding how it works, and then highlighting ways to make it, well . . . better.

A career in medicine is the birthing ground of unlimited stories. Not just hospital gossip, new and old, including jokes, aphorisms and anecdotes, but accounts of obscure and common diseases, unusual encounters and scenarios that remind us we are all mortal. For good measure I've woven in some bizarre historical tales which paint a slightly dubious and often unethical picture of medicine. After all, what is history if not the mistakes and errors from which you can learn vital lessons about life?

Before you cross the threshold, I must warn you. If you want a rose-tinted, sickly saccharine Panglossian view of the human body, then this book is not for you.

SAVE YOURSELF

Throughout each chapter, you'll also find 'Save Yourself' tips: practical hacks, advice and strategies to save yourself from your own body. I've no intention of reminding you to blink and breathe. By now, I would hope that you have nailed the fundamentals of staying alive. Even so, before we begin it's worth spelling out a select choice of lifestyle standards that will benefit your health across the board . . .

Diet

Diet is a huge part of any positive lifestyle change. Its constituents are hotly contested with no consensus reached on the 'best' approach, though you'd be wise to minimise processed foods as they're often high in sugar, salt and fat. I'm not going to promote any particular kind of healthy eating regime. Instead, let me cut to the chase by highlighting foods you should actively seek out and aim to consume often:

* **Plant foods** like vegetables, fruits, wholegrains, beans, nuts and seeds. These are nutrient-dense and also contain bioactive phytochemicals that are anti-inflammatory in nature.

* **Seafood** (if you eat fish that is), with a particular preference for oily fish like salmon, mackerel or sardines as they are rich in omega-3 fatty acids for good heart health.

* **Fermented foods** like Greek yoghurt, kimchi or sauerkraut, that promote beneficial bacteria in the gut, as well as **healthy fats** like unsaturated olive oil.

Ultimately, the best diet is one that you enjoy and makes you feel good. Eating cake and being healthy aren't mutually exclusive terms.

Hydration

Given that you're a walking bag of water, it should be common sense to say you need to stop yourself from drying out. When your body is deprived of water it steals water from other organs, including your brain, and that's . . . unwise.

Conversely, your body cannot cope with too much water. Your hypothalamus – the barometer in your brain – runs on a slight lag. So, it can take a while for your body to realise it has enough water in the tank. If you're very thirsty, and recklessly drink 5 litres of water in a short space of time, the cells will become overloaded with fluid. This results in a dilution of critical sodium levels; a potentially fatal condition known as hyponatremia.

All this just highlights how fragile your body can be. It can survive blizzards, beatings and even losing limbs, but under- or overwater it and you end up like that poor houseplant on your window ledge that seemed like a good idea at the time. In order to thrive, you should aim to consume about 2 litres over the course of each day.

Fitness

There is one magic pill that improves every facet of your health across the board. The only problem is you can't swallow this pill. Instead, you must endure it, or somehow make it enjoyable, and that pill is exercise.

Inactivity is a silent killer. The biggest evil modern society has gifted to us is a more sedentary lifestyle. Government guidelines for activity levels are typically mild and supposedly attainable. Just be honest and ask yourself how often do you get 150 minutes of moderate-intensity physical activity a week, let alone any strength activity?

All kinds of evidence exists to show that exercise can reduce the risk of early death. For one thing, you lose around 5 per cent of your muscle mass every decade after you cross the ripe old age of thirty. Yes, thirty. This rate of muscle loss doubles once you cross seventy, and is one of the central reasons why resistance training, promoting muscle strength, can make a massive difference to both quality of life and life expectancy. Ultimately, regular exercise of any kind benefits the mind as much as the body, and can be easily incorporated into a busy lifestyle. It really is the closest thing we have to real-life magic.

Alcohol and tobacco

Smoking and drinking aren't compulsory, and yet both pursuits are embedded in our culture. While the tide has been turning against tobacco for several decades now, it remains one of the single most damaging habits you can inflict on your body. Smokers not only have a reduced life expectancy, but they also experience proportionally more years of poor health than non-smokers. Besides outrageously raising the risk of lung cancer and various lung diseases, smoking ages you externally, from a yellowing of the teeth to thin, wrinkly skin. What's more, the chronic inflammation that results from smoking raises the risk of cardiovascular and neurodegenerative disease and on a cellular level causes cellular senescence, which literally means your cells become senile. On a brighter note, quitting can rapidly reduce all such risks to health, which makes it a no-brainer in my book.

If you think e-cigarettes and vaping are any healthier, think again. While we might still be accumulating the long-term risks of these newer tobacco alternatives, the data we have so far has confirmed numerous risks, from lung-related inflammation to full-blown lung failure – in some cases necessitating lung transplantation. Quite simply, if you want to keep your body from killing you then the only thing you should inhale is air.

Then we come to alcohol misuse, which is a significant threat to public health. Drinking excessively is associated with everything from heart and liver disease, digestive problems, weight gain and an increased risk of cancer. Quite simply, quitting – or even cutting down your intake – is one of the best things you can do to promote good health for life.

1. Is There a Plumber in the House?

EXPLORING GUT PIPES AND DIGESTIVE PROCESSES

IN MY VIEW OF HISTORY, more lives have been saved by the hand of plumbers than doctors. Surgeons, physicians and scientists get all the glory, but I feel it's time a chunk of that credit should go to that humble guild responsible for modern sanitation and sewage infrastructure. Why? Because a country's water system is directly linked to its population health. Without plumbers, deadly diseases like cholera would be rampant and there wouldn't be much point in saving for a pension.

Plumbers and doctors might seem like very different professions. When it comes to upholding public health, however, they're inextricably linked.

The body is a temple. That's the phrase we often trot out when it comes to wellness, but it couldn't be further from the truth. The fact is your body is a complex tower block with bespoke fittings, a series of overlapping drainage pipes, a sewage system with occasional backflows, many demanding tenants and even a few secret passageways. Steady now . . .

If we were presented with the blueprint for its construction, most people would take one look at the seemingly impenetrable tangle of plumbing and look around for someone in the trade to make sense of it. Which is where medics like me come in. If we're not on another job at the time.

Just as our ancestors eventually understood the benefits of civic sanitation, we can sometimes take a while to acknowledge the importance of keeping our human plumbing up to scratch. If your internal tubing sprouts a leak or a blockage point, it isn't just a question of a call out and a hit to the credit card. The consequences can be life-threatening.

Over time, I've come to view my purpose as a doctor to be more than just a dispenser of pills and potions. In my surgeon's gown and gloves, I might look like a civilised butcher but there's more to my role than that. Today, I think of myself as a mechanic for humans. A biomechanic if you will, and a tradesperson just like the plumber. In the same way that cars, buildings and tools need regular maintenance, the human body requires self-care and regular upkeep to avoid – or at least delay – misery, mishap and the morgue. With this in mind, let me take you on tour of the concealed pipes, service passageways and vents that form a central part of our anatomy, the gut.

Humble beginnings

Have you ever wondered how this all began? I don't mean philosophically but simply which of your body parts was first out of the blocks from the moment of egg fertilisation? Was it the brain? The heart? The backbone, or even the eyes? In answer, I would ask you to stop being such a poet about it, because the fact is that in that first magical moment you were nothing but an orifice indented on to a cluster of cells. That's right. You started life as an asshole.

Nobody can escape this unfortunate fact. We all kicked off in the same way, and it isn't pretty. The philosophers are allowed back in the room at this point, because of course this begs the question whether certain individuals every truly developed beyond this point.

Technically humans are deuterostomes. In other words, we belong to a group of animals whose blastopore (the first opening in the developing embryo) becomes its anus. Protostomes are animals whose blastopore becomes its mouth, but without exception we begin as bums, which is effectively the tail end of the gut. After the sperm breaks through the egg's outer membrane, the embryo splits into many different cells, eventually becoming a blastula. The blastula cells tear open from the inside out, forming an outlet called the blastopore, which, as you may have guessed, will one day develop into a glorious butthole (arguably blastopore is a far more sophisticated name for your rusty sheriff's badge, but for some reason it never caught on). Whatever you want to call it, the fact remains that your existence began as an embryonic, disconnected anus floating around in your mother's uterus, which is both a harsh truth and a highbrow insult if you ever care to use it.

With the blastopore now winking and floating happily in that amniotic sac, it widens and tunnels into the other side of the blastula where a mouth is formed. Yes, this is sounding like one of those horror films you regret watching midway through, but bear with me. By week six, that ass-to-mouth alien hybrid has evolved into something altogether more human. By then, you have developed the beginnings of your intestinal tracts inside the umbilical cord, the safety rope connecting you to the placenta. Mercifully, perhaps, your eyes only start developing at week eight. Until then, you're largely sheltered from the horrors of your own flesh twisting turning and mutating into an early version of what you are now. Traumatic stuff.

'You don't want to do it like that'

If you've ever built anything from scratch, like a robot monster made out of cereal packets (just me?), the early stages of construction rarely see it take on a form that resembles the final product. This is perfectly epitomised by the shape of your nascent embryological gut when you're a four-week-old human embryo. Through a series of elaborate origami-style folds, it transforms from a simple tube running up and down to an elaborate series of bulges and protrusions that include your liver, gall bladder, intestines, pancreas, oesophagus, mouth and stomach.

The one thing that always stumped me about embryology, and how our gut develops, is why it's doing what it does. How does it know the purpose of its existence? Take for example the small intestine. It loops around itself in our embryological bodies and journeys both inside and outside of the body. The mid-gut, which eventually consists of your small intestine, along with about half of your large intestine and your appendix, grows at a rapid pace. Such is the speed of development that at first it exceeds the capabilities of your primitive abdomen to contain it. Instead, these loops of intestine are exiled for a few weeks before snaking their way back in once your belly can contain them.

If any errors occur during this delicate dance, some babies can be born with an omphalocele, in which the intestines have developed in a sac outside the abdomen. This is frightening to see, even for a surgeon, who must attempt to rehouse it back where it belongs with immediate surgery. Then there are anorectal malformations that result in an underdeveloped anus and rectum that prevents normal stool passage; malrotation, when the intestines don't fold properly and are prone to twisting; and intussusception, in which the intestine retracts in on itself like a telescope causing bowel blockage. These are just scratching the surface of what can go wrong if just one element of the complex developmental choreography of the gut goes awry. It can result in lifelong health complications, and sometimes even death.

With all these various tubes, twists and turns you can see why I often talk about the gut in terms of plumbing. Known as the gastrointestinal system (or GI for short), it's one long and twisting pipe with valves, fittings and fixtures. It even boasts the functionality of a range of domestic appliances. What's more, the entire system is governed by what we now call a smart device.

Snack activation

When it comes to eating, guzzling down your meal deal is not as simple as draining bathwater into a down pipe. Yes, your lunch drops into a vertical tube once swallowed, but it's here that digestion takes place so your body can acquire energy from food, which makes it so much more complex than simply letting gravity take over. The path from mouth to anus is fraught with danger at every turn but also quite magical in the process, thanks to some bodging over the course of evolution that has resulted in a system that works.

The opening gambit of digestion is not marked by the moment that food hits your tongue. Those gears started turning long before you sat down to eat. Even when you poured the boiling water into your pot of instant noodles, releasing those sweet and sour aromas to seduce your nostrils, your digestive system was already activated. That trigger fired when the thought of a snack proved irresistible. As a result, a cascade of reflexes kicked off to stimulate the secretion of salivary juices, along with the production of more stomach acid and various enzymes in preparation for the feast.

The consumption of food, and the subsequent harvesting of fuel from it before the disposal of what's left over, is an act that is core to your well-being, which is why the gut was one of the first structures to develop when you were in the womb. From that blind, floating asshole in the moist environment of your mother's uterus a miracle took place.

Yes, you developed into a foetus, but more immediately you became a leech.

The umbilical cord is the safety rope that tethered you to your mother. It's the external plumbing system that doubled not only as your lifeline and source of food but a parasitical portal to the poor woman whose existence was set to revolve around you for quite some time to come. You enjoyed an idyllic existence in your amniotic sac, surrounded by fluid containing your own urine, free from the worries of metabolism and waste management. All your nutrients were conveniently provided to your door, nature's ultimate delivery service. The only cost was the discomfort you caused your provider for nine long months – until the terms of service changed.

At birth, and with the severing of your umbilical cord, your subscription came to an end. It's a rude awakening, and no wonder you cried. Why? Because from there on out you had to rely on your own pipework to carry out vital digestive and excretory functions. This was the moment that your inbuilt smart system came into play, priming your gut to eat, drink and evacuate your bowels on your own.

Down the hatch!

Your gut is active 24/7. It doesn't just wake up to allow you to shovel down food. It's also far more sophisticated than the trash masher you believe it to be. For example, when you're embarrassed, you don't just express this as a cherubic lighting up of the cheeks. The lining of your stomach also blushes and effectively looks to the floor. Scientists still have no idea what purpose this second-hand gastric awkwardness serves, but we know the gut doesn't stick purely to digestive duties. It isn't quite a sentient alien worm within the core of your body, performing a host of essential functions on your behalf, but as a concept it could help you to recognise the level of sophistication going on in there. Sweet dreams!

With this in mind, let me tell you that on some level your gut also serves as a second brain. This is down to the enteric nervous system, which, among the various other duties it performs, also flags when you're hungry and full up, in combination with the hunger hormones leptin (satiated) and ghrelin (hungry). It even has a role to play in being 'hangry' (that weird feeling of being on a short fuse in the absence of food). We all know there is a strong association between what you eat and how it makes you feel. In fact, all of us can nominate certain flavours that tap into our emotions and lift our spirits. Present me with a slice of banana cake and my personal storm clouds are guaranteed to part. This is not simply down to the association between food and memory but by virtue of the trillions of microbial colonisers that have conquered your gut and call it home.

The host with the most

Even locked in solitary confinement, we are never alone. The fact is we are outnumbered by the trillions of microscopic tenants living inside us all. Their kind has been in existence since the dawn of life on earth. They predate humans and will no doubt be around long after our light goes out.

We are, of course, talking about the bacterial population inside our gut, without whom we could not be ourselves. Collectively, these tiny organisms are called the microbiome. As far as we know, this is made up from around 4,000 different bacterial species. While their number is legion, their role for the most part is to keep you alive so they can thrive. In some ways you have an important part to play in this ecosystem. It is your job to keep them happy, and your welfare depends on it. Disrupt their delicate balance – which is easily done by leading an unhealthy lifestyle – and you could indirectly cause yourself all manner of problems, from autoimmune dysfunction to chronic bowel disease.

Nowadays we consider the field of microbiome science to be an area of modern research. The very first descriptions of 'little animals' or 'animalcules', that we now know as microbes like bacteria, parasites and various other single-celled organisms, date back to the seventeenth century. Then, the linen-drape making apprentice turned scientist Antonie van Leeuwenhoek used his handcrafted microscopes to examine the presence of these miraculous organisms from all manner of sources. In his quest to explore what was an undiscovered world at the time, van Leeunwenhoek observed the presence of bacteria on his own dental plaque and in the fluids sourced from his wife's body cavity after sex— sorry, research.

Often heralded as the father of microbiology, Antonie van Leeuwenhoek has the questionable honour of being the first human to see moving sperm cells. This certainly opened our eyes to the existence of the world within us. It's just since then we have shifted our focus into *what* role these microbes play, instead of just what *types* are present.

It has taken us close to four centuries to consider microbial communities as more than just pathogens. We now know that they have an intricate and essential role in determining the shape of our lives. This encompasses everything from training your immune system, influencing your behaviour through hormones and chemical releases, helping you to break down indigestible foods and even instilling us with some of their genes.

In recognising the relationship between microbes and humans, we would do well to stop thinking of ourselves as individuals and more as team members alongside an array of tiny organisms. The bacterial population of your microbiome serves a simple, life-saving role, which is to produce enzymes that ferment foods into short-chain fatty acids. Foods like bananas, beans, broccoli, cabbage and wholegrains are resistant to digestion in the small intestine. Moving into the large intestine, however, they are fermented or metabolised by the gut microbes to provide accessible carbohydrates. These little guys work their tails off, too. In your lifetime, they'll process around 35 tonnes of food.

Like any society, even if it is designed to be a utopia, errant rogues can linger in the darkness of the microbiome. One such malevolent critter of the bacterial underworld is *Clostridium difficile*; a bacterium that certainly instils even the hardiest healthcare worker with transient anal flutters and weak knees. It's responsible for diarrhoea and inflammation of the colon, often following extended antibiotic use (which in itself impacts the gut's health by wiping out large swathes of both good and bad gut bacteria and possibly skewing the internal battle in favour of the dark side).

Your relationship with both good and bad bacteria is complex but comes down to a simple truth: you only exist because they exist. Arguably, the gut's microbiome could be considered to be an entire forgotten organ system that is as critical for your survival as your beating heart.

The microbiome plays such a vital role in your survival that it also has the potential to influence brain development and behaviour. By releasing signalling molecules, your gut effectively talks with your central nervous system. With the microbiome acting as co-conspirator, it parleys with the brain via something known as the gut–microbiota–brain axis. These courier bugs send continuous messages back and forth along this inbuilt superhighway, which forms a pillar of what makes you human. Thanks to neurochemical transmitters, we're talking about a naturally occurring Bluetooth channel that allows two devices to pair and effectively function as one. This gut–brain set-up might not belt out Mariah Carey wherever you are in the house, but the two are in constant communication.

Community care

For all the wonders that we have discovered, the microbiome remains somewhat shrouded in mystery and mystique. This is mainly because our human brains have failed to unlock their secrets. What we do know is that the make-up of the population is somewhat dependent on our diet.

So how can we optimally care for this internal community of tiny creatures so they can be helpful companions? First of all, the microbiome craves diversity. This means eating many different types of food, particularly those of the plant variety, is essential. The oft-repeated dietary mantra, 'eat the rainbow' really does have some basis in science.

Your gut bacteria's favourite feast is fibre. Some (but not all) fibre is what's known as a prebiotic, which provides your gut bacteria with helpful nutrients so they can thrive. Your bacteria also love gorging on molecules called polyphenols, which you can find in things like blueberries, extra virgin olive oil and even dark chocolate. These foods effectively keep a healthy gut biome in good shape. Foods like yoghurt, kefir, sourdough bread and even some cheese often contain live bacteria, aka probiotics. Fermented foods like miso, kimchi and sauerkraut are often referred to as postbiotics as they encourage gut bacteria to produce useful molecules such as fatty acids. Ultimately, a balanced, healthy diet will ensure that you have all three 'biotic bases' covered.

Finally, a word on things that make your gut bugs less happy. A diet very high in red meat and particularly those reliant on ultra-processed foods can upset the microbiome. The reasons are not yet fully understood, but it's thought that certain gut bacteria release harmful chemical compounds after being exposed to red meat in the digestive tract. When consumed in excess, this can cause inflammation in the body which affects biome balance. Of course, life is about moderation. Your gut bugs cannot expect a diet free from the occasional caramel crème donut, but it should be part of a healthy, balanced diet. We often say that something is 'good for you'. What we really mean is that it's good for your gut microbiome. Keep those internal squatters happy, and they'll look after the place for you.

Food for thought

As a high school student studying biology, I was always perplexed by the subject of digestion. It confused me even more at medical school when I learned that it was even more complex than I'd been taught. With my nose in medical textbooks, I discovered the passage of food through the body was spectacularly nuanced and demanded the coordination of precise and delicate processes. It wasn't until I saw them for myself, as a surgeon wrist-deep in wriggling intestines, that I realised digestion is the furnace through which we light the fire to drive functions essential for life. I have even come to think of the gut as the centrepiece of the body, although the heart and brain may argue this point.

At its most reductionist level, digestion involves consuming our external environment to build our internal one. We feed in everything from gases (air), liquids (tea) and solids (burgers), extract what we need to survive and then neatly discard the waste product. We assume all of this takes place inside us, hidden away from prying eyes, like the Oompa Loompas that keep the Wonka factory ticking. But what if I said that your intestines and the process of digestion is not inside you, but outside?

Granted, it's an unusual concept to grasp but the digestive system isn't really inside us. We are just so intricately folded and formed that the length of gut that meanders from mouth to anus is no more than a deep groove from one external aperture to another. It's a member of the outside world that transits through us and we are simply a conduit that facilitates it, like a purpose-built tunnel for an underground train line.

The art of digestion – less Leonardo and more Pollock – involves consuming the outside to turn it into an inside. This is introspection at its most guttural level. What we are right now, our physical form, is a by-product of digestion. Ultimately, it's an unintended but welcome side effect of a long, coordinated series of sickeningly complex biochemical reactions and equations.

In reality, there is no distinct line between the inside and out. On a cultural, social and sexual level, however, we've attempted to obsessively disown our delicate inner workings. From the cacophony of groans, moans and burps, the natural symphonic embouchure created by the windpipe orchestra down below, to the various aromas exuding from our exit orifices, these are the sounds and smells we have strived to hide and disown for centuries. Do you smell that? Wasn't me.

Every hint of this beast below deck that we call digestion can occasionally confuse, embarrass or even frighten us. We've even attempted to exterminate and systematically eradicate any sign of its good work by means of sweet-smelling lotions, deodorising sprays, scented wipes and ventilation systems. It is a basic human instinct for us to want to control our environment; naturally, this extends to our internal ecosystem. As a society, we have effectively launched a guerrilla campaign to remove any evidence and trace of the twisting tube of foreignness we are wrapped around. Our mission is to cleanse ourselves from all the associated smells, sounds and visual outpourings – sometimes from both ends – that have come to horrify us so acutely.

A HITCHHIKER'S GUIDE TO THE GUT

Now we know that the microbiome plays a major role in governing your gut, like a legion of micro-plumbers in charge of the internal piping, let's explore the range of appliances through which food is processed once it drops into the system. At the top end, your mouth chews everything you toss into it like a high-end food waste disposer. Duly crunched and crushed, you then gulp it down into your oesophagus, or food pipe. Then, in the depths of the stomach, the pulverised food boluses are mixed with stomach juices, not unlike a washing machine in the middle of a spin cycle. Admittedly, you might not want clothes treated quite in this way, especially when your stomach adds acid to the mixture. This helps to break down food, but it wouldn't do much for your delicates.

Next up – courtesy of the pancreas and gall bladder – you have digestive enzymes, which are basically high-end laundry detergents without the commercial packaging. They contain amylase to break down starch, protease to pulverise proteins and lipase to take care of those greasy stains known as fats.

By the time your food emerges from your small intestine, where this somewhat hardcore wash cycle has taken place, it looks like a very thin and unappetising soup. Here, it finds an ever-hungry recipient ready and waiting to take over the next stages. Your colon performs a crucial function in providing the final rinse and dry cycle. As well as reabsorbing water and electrolytes, it's the breeding ground for the majority of your microscopic tenants. This is where they do their dirty business by fermenting and breaking down various foods to release essential nutrients, before making a chocolate deposit in the bank of rectum. (Feel free to break here and grab a snack before we continue.)

The gut is one of the most underrated organs in the human body. Arguably it's not really one organ but four. We're talking about the stomach along with the small and large intestine, all of which tend to get more press than the lesser-known mesentery; a yellow, fatty, fan-shaped structure that houses the blood supply to the gut. The mesentery is such an underappreciated organ it was only bestowed the title 'organ' in 2017. Without it, the gut would have no power. If we're being greedy, we can even dare to consider the gall bladder, liver, pancreas and oesophagus to be part of the same gut family. Ultimately, these adjacent structures are all inexorably linked to the factory line that is the digestive process.

All mouth

If the soul resided in the gut, the mouth would be the window. We can do a lot with our mouths, but my favourite of its roles is eating.

Thankfully it's ably supported by a crescendo of saliva, a regiment of teeth and a serpentine muscular structure called the tongue, which can destroy almost any foreign invader that sets foot inside. Your mouth is also host to a hidden army of bacteria; these form your oral microbiome, a protective front that contributes to your oral health.

The mouth is the first line of defence; taking the bite out of the enemy's initial assault. Chewing might seem like a chore, but it means less work for your stomach and reduces the chances of indigestion and bloating.

To aid the chewing process, among other things, glands in your mouth secrete a clear fluid called saliva. You might spit it out in an expression of disgust or in anger, but ultimately it's triggered when we're hungry or pick up on the thought, sight or smell of food we fancy. Saliva doesn't just lubricate the mouth as you prepare to gorge on food; it also contains small amounts of hydrogen peroxide, which can kill bacteria. You've been warned: your mouth uses chemical warfare tactics.

What's more, it contains analgesic compounds that are stronger than any drug I can prescribe you. So, if you have a sore throat, you may find that eating something, or simply just chewing gum, to stimulate the production of pain-busting chemical infused saliva, may ease your symptoms. In fact, saliva even contains an ingredient similar to that found in pee. Urea helps to balance the acid/alkaline (PH) level of your oral cavity in order to protect your teeth. It's a truly multifunctional fluid, but its most important contents are all the salivary enzymes, which can help to break down food.

Your oral microbiome, backed up by saliva, plays a central role in determining the smell of your breath. Even if you're relatively healthy, no doubt you've woken up in the morning and wondered why the people you love are grimacing to your face. For the most part, the pungent odours on your breath are produced by bacteria that feed on decomposing food. For example, the chemicals putrescine (as in to putrefy) and cadaverine (as in cadaver) literally smell like decay and death. It's not something you want to detect on someone, and equally it might explain why you may have gone into work to find an exclusion zone in place around you.

Swallowing for science

I remember the first time I took a thin flexible telescope with a light attached and passed it deep into a patient's throat. With great care, as I did as a child playing the classic battery-powered board game, Operation, I guided the instrument down the oesophagus to the stomach and even to the first part of the small intestine. I marvelled at how delicate the internal linings were, aware that any incorrect movement of my scope could cause pain or even puncture the linings. Sometimes in medicine, however, the benefits of performing a procedure far outweigh the small risks if by chance we identify the cause of a patient's reflux disease or pick up a cancer or growth in the early stages.

Back in the nineteenth century, when much of the digestive system was still open to exploration, pioneering physicians were a little freer and easier when it came to taking risks in the name of medical science. It was a German physician named Adolf Kussmaul who built a tube with mirrors containing a small lamp so that he could peer into the tract that links the mouth to the stomach. Aware that the gag reflex could scupper his exploration, Kussmaul ingeniously hired a sword swallower to test out his new device. It opened up an inside view of the oesophagus, proving to be an early design for what we now know as an endoscope: a small camera that helps doctors to look inside your guts.

Ode to the oesophagus

In the same way that worms use waves of contracting muscles to slither along the ground, your digestive system employs the same basic process to shuttle food along. This is known as peristalsis. It happens when there's an alternating sequence of muscle contraction and relaxation, like a Mexican wave passing through a crowd at the stadium. This is how food is driven along your pipe. Thankfully, the process is independent of gravity, which is why you can still swallow food and drink if you're hanging upside down. It's just not recommended.

If you do attempt this, let's not forget that the human body is always a breath away from catastrophe. One of the first pitfalls of your gastrointestinal system greets you at the upper end. As bad designs go, it's potentially award-winning, and boils down to the fact that your food pipe (the oesophagus) is fitted right next to your air pipe (the trachea). It also shares the same entrance (the pharynx), which covers all the space from the nose to your voice box (the larynx). To ensure food and drink doesn't take a detour into the lungs via the breathing pipe, you've got a tiny flap of tissue (the epiglottis), which closes the opening to the trachea whenever you swallow. So, if you're with friends, eating, talking and laughing at the same time, food can easily take a wrong turn, slip into your airways and then bring silence to the entire restaurant as you choke until your eyeballs bulge.

Nobody experiences this more acutely than babies who choke on a regular basis. I'm reliably informed that babies are quite important to the survival of our species, so how did we end up with this kind of dodgy set-up?

This sometimes-fatal quirk is an evolutionary trade-off, a necessary evil. The fact is the larynx is low down in our throats as it enables us to vocalise and produce complex speech much better than it if was located higher up. As a result, it competes for space with our food pipes, and throws a risk into the mix that if you get it wrong you might die.

If we wanted to renegotiate this 2-for-1 piping arrangement and design a human with separate orifices for eating and breathing, we would have to sacrifice all the wonderful things that go into being human. Talking, singing and shouting at the BMW driver who cut you up: all these simple pleasures would have to go just so that we could stuff our faces without risk of choking. There are alternative arrangements, of course. Birds, for example, have a decent gap between their windpipes and oesophagus, which means they don't fall off a branch mid-song having accidentally inhaled a worm. The trouble is that whenever you move two orifices apart, you have to move another two closer together. In humans, if we wanted to talk and eat without risk of choking this would mean we'd have to live like our winged friends with a cloaca, also known as a common exhaust pipe for urine and faeces. It's worth noting that squids have it far worse. Food passes through their brains, which strikes me as quite a high price to pay for the chance to breathe without risk of choking on a baguette. In this view, maybe just be careful next time you boast about your new park run PB while still wrestling with a mouthful of pasta.

Save yourself

I don't need to spell out why a blocked airway isn't a good look. Or perhaps I do. Even brief shortages in oxygen supply to the brain can be deleterious. Usually, the body reflexively flaps around like a fish out of water, spluttering, coughing and gagging in a desperate attempt to clear the offending morsel of food which dared to enter the wrong tunnel. Should you find yourself in the presence of someone turning puce in the face, there are several ways that you can establish your reputation as a hero.

The Heimlich manoeuvre was named after its creator, medical maverick and thoracic surgeon, Dr Henry Heimlich. For decades after its inception, many people believed that it was the only way to save someone who was choking, due in no small part to Hollywood-produced versions of this simple act being shown to miraculously save lives. The Heimlich can help, but it's certainly not the only option. It may not even be the best one on the table, or the floor, depending on where your victim is floundering.

Repeated blows (or 'blocks') using the heel of your hand between someone's shoulder blades is an equally effective initial option. It's arguably much less violent than bear hugging a choking victim, especially if they're elderly. Most emergency choking protocols now recommend five back blocks. Should that fail to fix the problem then perform five abdominal thrusts (previously known as the Heimlich manoeuvre) by placing a hand around someone's mid abdomen and thrusting inwards and upwards. If the victim continues to choke, call the emergency services.

Shut that door!

Towards the end of your food pipe, there's a single-flow valve that really could be more foolproof called the lower oesophageal sphincter. It connects your oesophagus and stomach, and it's the first of your sphincters to feel the punishment of those fiery hot wings and the backsplash of stomach acid. If excess stomach acid repeatedly bubbles back through this valve, it burns the living hell out of your oesophagus, usually sometime around 4am. Sometimes this sphincter can be a bit janky, like a door that doesn't close properly and lets the draught in. If this is the case, it isn't a breeze you get but what can feel like the tendrils of hell.

A taste of stomach acid

In the stewing pit that is the stomach, engulfed by torrents of saliva, mucus and acids and whipped ferociously by undulating waves of muscular contractions, your food is churned into chyme – a semi-solid, partially digested paste.

In the nineteenth century, scientists disagreed about how the stomach worked. Some hypothesised that it was a mechanical sequence in which the muscular contractions ground up the food. Others thought it was a chemical process, while a few dared to suggest it could be a mixture of both. Oddly enough, the question was answered thanks to arguably one of the most unethical experiments in the history of medicine.

In 1822 a Canadian fur trapper named Alexis St. Martin was accidentally shot by a stray musket. The blast left a fist-sized hole in the middle of his abdomen. By rights, it should have killed him. Thanks to the efforts of army surgeon William Beaumont, however, the victim survived. St. Martin lived to trap another day, and yet the wound failed to close and heal. Instead, an abnormal connection between the skin and stomach formed, known as a gastric fistula. Dr Beaumont discovered that in the right light he could peer through this natural aperture and observe his patient's stomach in action. It was, the doctor realised, an opportunity to observe digestion in real time, a literal window to the inner workings of this previously mysterious process.

Over the next decade, Dr Beaumont formed a morally dubious working relationship with his human fishbowl. It was one that enabled him to perform a series of experiments. Somehow, he persuaded poor Alexis St. Martin to swallow different kinds of food attached to string. This allowed the doctor to peer through the fistula and watch the digestive process with his own eyes before hauling out the remains for analysis. He was even said to have popped his tongue through the fistula to determine the astringent but magical properties of stomach fluids. It was through these abhorrent and mostly disgusting experiments that Doctor Beaumont was able to deduct that our digestive juices consisted of mucus enzymes and acid.

One of the most important parts of the digestive juices produced by the stomach is hydrochloric acid. This potent chemical cocktail is powerful enough to strip the rust off metal. In your stomach, it can kill harmful bacteria while playing a central role in the digestive process. So, what's stopping it from burning through the stomach wall and liquifying us from the inside? The answer is mucus. This stuff coats the stomach lining, forming a protective wall against the acid. Thankfully, the mucus tends to have the upper hand. When it loses the odd battle, the outcome can be painful and takes the form of stomach ulcers.

Through a combination of science and meddling, we've found ways to turn our bodies against themselves. NSAIDS, which stands for non-steroidal anti-inflammatory drugs, are a case in point. This common over-the-counter medicine is often branded as ibuprofen, and acts on pain by reducing the production of the pain-signalling molecule prostaglandin. It does this by blocking an enzyme called COX-2 and can be very effective. However, one other function of prostaglandin is to reduce stomach acid and increase mucus production to provide natural regulation of the stomach lining. Taking large doses of ibuprofen, or taking it over a long period of time, can result in ulcer formation (effectively a hole in the stomach) – something I hate dealing with as a surgeon because of the pain and suffering it causes the patient, as well as the potential to kill them.

We know that the mucus wall can also be compromised by a bacterium called *Helicobacter pylori*, allowing the acid to burn through. For a long time, however, scientists wrongly linked ulcers to stress or spicy food. In the 1980s, it was Dr Barry Marshal who set the world straight by deliberately ingesting the bacteria he suspected of being responsible to induce severe gastritis (a precursor to the formation of stomach ulcers). This experiment on himself caused Dr Marshal both intense pain and copious vomiting, but it also enabled him to take a sample of his own gut to prove the bacteria was present and responsible. As bacteria can be easily treated with a course of antibiotics, Dr Marshal recovered to publish his findings and went on to win a Nobel Prize for his efforts.

Intestine times

When your stomach has finished beating your ready meal into chyme, it's time for this delightful mixture to make its way to the doorway to the small intestine. This is also called the pylorus, which is Latin for 'gatekeeper'.

It takes around ninety minutes for 50 per cent of the contents of the stomach to empty into the small intestine. For this reason, it's usually a good idea to avoid eating in the two to three hours before you go to bed. It means you're not sleeping with a full stomach as this can cause indigestion and potentially wreak havoc on your sleep.

A decent kip might be even harder to find if you've made room for that dessert. Have you ever wondered why you always have room for one even after a particularly satisfying meal? Well, the tales of the second stomach are true.

Just as your mouth is fitted with taste buds, so your stomach also has taste receptors. These can recognise the value of certain foods and teach us to seek them out. We can thank our predecessors for this ancestral reflex, as in times of famine a sweet food represented an energy-dense and high-value commodity. As a result, when you're presented with a sugary delight, it can trigger your stomach's taste receptors to produce the hunger hormone, ghrelin. This waistline-undermining agent can override your brain's signals that previously told you that you were full and urge you to stock up before famine hits. Next time you're presented with that irresistible treacle pudding, even though you're full to burst, it could be your second stomach that puts paid to your resolve. You can blame your biology.

Hold my hair back

The journey through the digestive tract is usually one way; occasionally, however, things don't quite go to plan and some contents make their way back up the pipe.

Nausea is one of the most insidious symptoms. From an evolutionary point of view, it's your body's way of signalling that you're poisoned. Your body also tends to give due warning, which is all part of the unpleasant process that can result in vomiting. An early sign that you're about to be sick is an increase in saliva production, known as water brash. Basically, your body that knows you're about to force the acidic content of your stomach into your mouth, and it wants to protect your tooth enamel. Think of it as an inbuilt act of self-care.

Save yourself

More often than not, if the stomach needs to reject its contents you're effectively just a bystander. In some cases, however, the feelings associated with nausea can be managed. Ginger is known to contain anti-nausea properties, mainly due to the less than ingeniously named chemical gingerol, and many people find that chewing on ginger sweets or even ginger root can ease the symptoms. It does this by increasing the rate at which your stomach empties into the small intestine (increased gastric emptying).

If your nausea is due to motion sickness then consider your vision to be key to steadying the ship. Why? Because when there is a mismatch between your eyes and balance sensors the brain can interpret it as poisoning. When travelling by a means beyond your control (such as on a ship or as a car passenger) the key is to keep your eyes fixed on the horizon. This lessens the discord between what you're feeling and what you're seeing, which helps the eyes and balance sensors coordinate their information better. To that end, if you do struggle with motion sickness, try sitting at the front of the ride to take in as much horizon as possible.

A moment of bile

As the food transits into the first part of the small intestine – assuming you haven't thrown up from that extra portion of pudding – it's greeted by digestive aids and enzymes produced by three fascinating organs. The gall bladder and pancreas provide vital functions, but they're dwarfed by the beast lurking in the abdominal cavity. We're talking about that hepatic hulk, the monster of metabolism, the abdominal abomination . . . the liver.

Whatever you put into your body, even sometimes if it borders on idiocy, the liver metabolises the lot, which is shorthand for converting what you feed it into energy. It laughs in the face of your favourite celebrity influencer's detox products because it can tackle more toxins in a minute than a lifetime of juice cleanses. The digestive system sends all the nutrients to this mega factory. There, in among its many departments, the liver breaks down fat and extracts energy, while also churning out proteins, hormones and clotting factors that stop you bleeding out from a cut.

Putting a precise figure on the number of functions the liver performs is a running challenge for scientists, but we're looking at at least 500. It's so complex that no machine can replicate its function. The only fix for a broken liver (which we often call liver failure) is getting a new one by transplant. Like Doctor Who, its powers of regeneration are so incredible that as surgeons we don't need to replace them very often. Even when it's necessary, you can donate 70 per cent of your liver to someone and it'll grow into a fully functioning model, while yours will return to normal in just a couple of months.

While it's fair to say that without a liver we'd be in a dreadful mess, it's an organ responsible for producing the hideous green fluid that is vital for breaking down fats in your food. Like a serial killer might keep a vat of acid in the garage, bile is the body's disposal liquid of choice. The liver is such a prodigious producer of this digestive juice that much is sent to storage in its sidekick organ, the gall bladder.

Bile basically contains acids and salts that emulsify fats. The gall bladder does a great job of serving as a lock-up facility for the liver . . . until it fails when you need it most. At medical school, I spent many hours in the dissection rooms marvelling at this quirky anatomy. In every cadaver I opened up, the basic gall bladder was always the same and yet there was incredible variation in the structure of the bile pipes. These flowed from the liver and connected to the gall bladder and small intestine. The gall bladder really is one of the most variable parts of human anatomy, and it's for this reason that removing one from a patient can be so fraught with danger. In fact, studies have shown that damage to the common bile duct, which connects the liver to the small intestine, can cost a patient up to a decade of life.

I've had so many run-ins with rogue gall bladders that I have formed a love–hate relationship with them. At best, they ensure the digestive system continues to break down the evidence of your food crimes throughout your life. At worst, it's nothing more than a primitive storage sack in which tiny balls of cholesterol or bilirubin can form and make your life a misery.

About 10 per cent of the population develop gallstones in their gall bladder. Fortunately, very few experience symptoms, but some of those that do can wish for the sweet release of death. Gallstones have become an increasingly major pathology due to the excesses of our modern lives. Overeating and a diet high in fat and cholesterol can increase the chances of them forming. Gallstones, like rock solid caviar, can shift into the gall bladder ducts and ultimately block the flow of bile, causing inflammation and pain that can quickly escalate.

This is what I hate about gall bladders because a blocked duct can cause a patient untold misery. The organ is designed to contract around mealtimes, squeezing out bile, but just imagine if that sack is loaded with stones? The patient soon becomes terrified of teatime.

For very different reasons, removing a gall bladder is one of the most satisfying operations, both for patient and surgeon. It can spell an instant end to pain and discomfort if you're in possession of one that's gone rogue. It's also such a common complaint that it provides me with steady work.

The fun and games aren't always restricted to the gall bladder. Occasionally a gallstone can wander out, travel down a forbidden path and lodge itself near the pancreas. This is an equally important organ, which produces digestive enzymes. If some adventurous gallstones find themselves near the pancreas they can block the flow of enzymes, so they essentially start attacking the pancreas itself. This is known as pancreatitis, which is your body's way of reminding you that it has the capacity to be a Hannibal Lector to your inner Clarice Starling. Worryingly, pancreatitis can have a mortality rate of up to 1 per cent.

What can we say about the pancreas? For starters, not many people even realise it exists. We're talking about something in the recesses of your abdomen that looks like an inedible mini corn on the cob. People only really take notice of the pancreas when it doesn't do one of the few jobs it is tasked with, which includes the production of insulin. It also becomes the focus of attention when it attempts to kill you by stealth. Pancreatic cancer has one of the worst survival rates because symptoms don't often present until it's too late. It's like discovering that a disgruntled employee has been quietly sabotaging the business while pretending to be productive.

When we consider all the problems that can occur with bile storage, perhaps we should review our love affair with the liver and ask why it can't just produce the appropriate amount instead of sometimes making more than required. It's a good question, but then the answer is similar to one given by the water board when asked why we need a reservoir. Storage matters, because ultimately it's about delivery on demand.

Save yourself

If you have gall bladder issues, stick to a low-fat diet. This makes sense, as it reduces the need for the organ to contract and squeeze out a load of fat-emulsifying bile. Should you be unlucky enough to develop gallstones, the last thing you want is a gall bladder that's pulling tight all the time. The pain can be excruciating, and even dietary modifications are simply a temporary measure for most people – the only way to 'cure' gall bladder woes is to have it removed.

Reappraising the appendix

When I first saw a real-life appendix, attached to the first part of the colon and fluttering in the crevice of the abdomen, I immediately thought of how this worm-like structure almost killed my cousin all those years ago. Just because it tried to take out a family member, however, I should be objective in my appraisal. It's believed the appendix plays an important role in repopulating the microbiome of the bowel, acting as a sort of storage tank for good bacteria. This is important if you suffer from any kind of diarrhoeal illness. Throughout history, this has often been down to unsanitary conditions, but I dare say some TikTok Laxative Challenge might be just as culpable today. Whatever the cause, a case of the shits can deplete the bowel of bacteria. While we can survive and even thrive without an appendix, it's believed that it can serve as a means of restoring the good stuff.

Eau de colon

When I'm opening up a patient's abdomen during major surgery, the intestines look like particularly well-soaked and enlarged udon noodles, but for giants. It never ceases to amaze me how such a long tube can be forced into twists and loops inside a cavity that can barely contain it. The small intestine is nested in the middle of the belly. It's about 20 to 25 feet long, but we'd need a microscope to view its full extent. This is because the interior is fitted with loads of tiny finger-like projections called villi. These projections have even smaller projections called microvilli, which collectively increase the surface area available for absorption. This all makes perfect sense because about 90 per cent of our food is absorbed in the small intestine. Food travels through this section at just 6 inches per hour, which is markedly slower that the rate at which you wolfed it down.

After most of the contents of the food are absorbed in the small intestine, the remaining contents move on to the large intestine. Think of this section as the body's sewage pipe. Crucially, water and salts are reabsorbed here, before the final waste product is ready to make its way back into the world.

Defecation nation

Over the course of a lifetime, your intestines can handle around 11,000kg of poo, which is about the same weight as a hefty elephant. At any time in your adult life, your digestive tract contains a few kilos of the stuff, which means you are literally full of shit.

In my fifth month as a first-year doctor, while on a surgical rotation, I was on call with my registrar, or senior doctor. Surgical registrars are frightening creatures that inspire shock, awe and terror wherever they go. I can say this as I've been a registrar for many years, although try as I might I have never lived up to expectation. On my rounds, I saw an elderly male patient with a swollen, distended abdomen. It made the poor guy appear nine months pregnant, and I really hoped that I could help. So, I began by percussing his abdomen like you would a drum. The sound it made was hollow, suggesting it was full of gas.

I suspected he might have a sigmoid volvulus. Elderly patients are at higher risk for this particular condition in which a part of the large intestine – the sigmoid colon – twists on itself. It's particularly dangerous because if it stays twisted for a long period of time it can cause increasing pain, or worse, a compromise to the blood supply and bowel death. This needs prompt untwisting or 'decompression'.

With trepidation I approached my registrar and shared my assessment of the patient. When I asked what I should do, he looked at me as if to mock my lack of knowledge. 'You need to use a flatus tube,' he told me. 'Look it up and let me know when you've done it.'

This was particularly daunting as I'd never seen one inserted before. All I knew was that it's a plastic tube inserted into the patient's derriere to encourage free-flowing movement inside the colon.

In desperation I searched YouTube videos on how to perform the procedure, grabbed the flatus tube from the stock room and then headed to see the patient with more doubt than determination. That day I was wearing a smart blue shirt and chinos. This will become relevant later, unfortunately.

As per the instructions I'd picked up online, I positioned the patient in a foetal position and inserted the small plastic tube into his back passage. At first . . . well, nothing. So, I advanced the tubing slightly more, only to be greeted by a squeal of agony from the patient followed by the loud hiss of pungent sulphur-infused gas as it invaded the room. Just as I drew breath to toast our success, I was unceremoniously blasted with a brown liquid as it sprayed through the tubing in my grasp.

I froze, anxious to mask my revulsion from the patient, just as my registrar walked in. His expression matched my own, but quicky turned to glee.

'Rule number one of surgery club,' he said, keeping his distance while my patient breathed a sigh of relief. 'Always point the tube towards the most junior person in the room.'

'Understood,' I said, somewhat traumatised.

'Rule number two,' he added. 'If you'd prefer me not to think of you as a cretin then attach the tube to a bag before insertion.'

A POTTED HISTORY OF POOING

Pooing is the end game for the digestive process, but thankfully not in a constant, steady trickle. Even when it's fully functioning, everyone has a unique evacuation rate, so don't be comparing bowel-movement frequency with co-workers. Save that for the retirement home.

The phrase nothing is certain except death and taxes is incomplete. Shitting is also an inevitability, and nobody is above it. Wherever you're seated in the banqueting hall, from the top table to the servant's bench, whatever you eat comes out in the same form. It's also one of those subjects that's still considered taboo, which is unhelpful from a health practitioner's perspective. People are either reluctant to come forward with concerns, or simply unaware of warning signs of an underlying issue because the facts aren't part of the national conversation. So, as a public service, let me take you on a journey through the tunnels of mystery and medicine to bring our lavatory habits out into the light.

Societies, religions and cultures have long tried to present the act of defecation as humanity's dirty little secret. In my own experience, when I went to visit family in India in the early nineties, I would see people subjugated into handling human excrement by hand and cleaning public latrines under dire conditions. These people, a group known as Dalits, were the unfortunate victims of the horrifically backward caste system, where the lowly placed 'untouchables' were for many centuries forced by society to handle the waste of those higher up in the hierarchy. Sometimes, shit really does roll downhill.

Oppression aside, the one thing that can make anyone feel like a king or queen, regardless of social standing, is their own porcelain throne. From royal chamber pots to communal outhouses and holes in the ground, technological advances have spawned the modern, seated, flushable toilet – a seat fit for reflection and a moment away from the stresses of modern life. The modern toilet, a transition point between human intimacy and architectural greatness, while alleviating many of the diseases that flourished with poor sanitation and open public defecation, has also given rise to haemorrhoids, bowel conditions like diverticulosis, and even constipation – the scourge of every strainer in town. What's less commonly recognised is that such afflictions tend to affect those of us in the western world due to our love of supposedly 'civilised' toilets.

You can blame the lure of the seat for this modern-day health crisis. Why? Because the position in which you settle in order to do your business can result in high pressures being exerted on the end of the gut. This increased internal pressure results in a 'blow out' causing either balloon-like hernias to form in the colon (known as diverticular disease) or the appearance of swollen, juicy veins that line your anus (fondly known as haemorrhoids, or piles).

What happens when you poo?

Have you ever sat down and wondered how your body coordinates a bowel motion? Exactly what goes on in there that triggers a poo? Well, even the most primitive things sometimes require extraordinary sophistication to produce.

This simple sounding process requires all manner of bodily tensions, dilations and contractions. It's a masterclass of contortions driven at first by instinct, so it seems somehow mean-spirited of us to dismiss the act as merely 'taking a dump'.

On its final descent from the end of the colon to the rectum, faecal matter shifts a gear and drives forward, clearing folds of rectal tissue like the *Millennium Falcon* on a flight through a planetary chasm. As the rectal chamber enlarges and fills with what is the final evolution of food, stretch receptors in the walls of the rectum alert us that it might be time to spill some beans. In response, the internal and external anal sphincters begin their eternal tug of war. The internal pushing for an exit, the external holding back the brown tide until decorum can be achieved.

Despite what appears to be opposing roles, both sphincters are tied by destiny. Like yin and yang, one cannot exist without the other, and you will be thankful for that. The internal anal sphincter serves no master except basic, barbaric and crude reflexes and represents the unconscious mind. The external anal sphincter is your indentured servant, who obeys your brain's command and gives you voluntary sphincter control.

When the time is right, the two will combine effectively to allow the floodgates to open.

It's a blessing that you're fitted with a mechanism that allows you to discriminate between letting out a fart and a full blown poo. Like some kind of shitting superpower, the rectoanal inhibitory reflex (RAIR) (also known as the anal sampling mechanism, anal sampling reflex, rectosphincteric reflex, or anorectal sampling reflex) can detect if the package knocking at the back door is solid or gaseous in nature. Ultimately, your RAIR allows you to blow off safely even if a poo is also imminent. You can't put a price on that.

However, even the most well calibrated of instruments can wobble. This reflex isn't foolproof when it comes to distinguishing between liquid and gas. So, when you're having one of those days when your bowels are running more than you are, don't tempt fate by trusting a fart unless you're sitting comfortably with your buttocks a few inches above shallow water. Sharting in public is undeniably one of the most miserable feelings one can experience (so I'm told).

Anyone who claims they don't fart is a liar. It's part of the digestive process, and is a result of swallowing air with our food (as nobody dines in a vacuum). We all do it, and even if we try to hold it in that body gas will find its way out. Whether the leak is so small that nobody can detect it, or you're the kind of person to make a song and dance out of it, us humans pass an average of fourteen farts a day. Each bottom burp mostly consists of odourless gases like hydrogen, nitrogen and carbon dioxide. It's just there's also a very small component called hydrogen sulphide, and that packs an olfactory punch. With a bouquet like rotten eggs, this is the chemical responsible for that nasty niff. While some people have intestinal gas that also contains methane, the fact is, it's a chemical compound that has no sweet finish on the fragrance front or any odour at all.

While the external anal sphincter is under voluntary control, which means you know the difference between a poo and a fart, the internal anal sphincter is involuntary. In extremes of age (infants and occasionally the very elderly), defecation occurs by reflex action without the voluntary control of the external anal sphincter. Loss of control – called faecal incontinence – may also be caused by physical injury, nerve injury, constipation, diarrhoea, loss of storage capacity in the rectum, intense fright, inflammatory bowel disease, psychological or neurological factors, childbirth or death.

Assuming you're in control but not in a position to act upon the urge, let's say because you're midway through twenty lengths of the public swimming pool, then the material in the rectum is often returned to the colon by reverse peristalsis. There, more water is absorbed into the faeces, which is stored until the next mass peristaltic movement of the transverse and descending colon.

When the time and place comes to poo, you perform a Valsalva manoeuvre. It's not a conscious move, like the floss dance, but more of an intuitive urge to push. By exhaling against a closed airway, often described as straining, you increase the pressure inside the abdomen. In turn the pelvic floor muscles relax, the perineum descends and the external anal sphincter opens up, delivering your creation into the world.

All strain, no gain

Due to their extra internal organs like ovaries and a uterus, females have slightly longer and more tortuously winding colons than males. Lady poo chutes can also be less muscular. As muscle helps to push contents through, this makes women more prone than men to constipation. We're talking about a common condition in which it feels difficult to poo. While everyone empties their bowels at different rates, you could be said to be constipated if you fail to go less than three times in a week.

To fight the good fight against constipation, the ingenuity of humans has given us laxatives. Some soften the stool by allowing it to retain more water and these are known as osmotic laxatives. Others help them to become more water-absorbent and easier to pass – these are called bulk-forming agents. In addition, stimulant laxatives help the gut in its contractions while enemas are a form of laxative that enter battle through the back passage.

While laxatives may help both men and women with the occasional bouts of constipation, they are not a cure but a quick fix. The fact is laxatives can put stress on your digestive system and the microbes that live in there. Overuse can even impact gut function by weakening the intestinal muscles and nerve response, thus leaving you hooked on laxatives to maintain bowel function, so use them with respect. In fact, some stimulant laxatives like sennoside, if used prodigiously and chronically, can paint the walls of your colon such that it resembles leopard print. Louis Vuitton colons, although harmless, are not in vogue.

The causes of constipation are widespread, but it often boils down to toilet habits. The nerves of the gut are closely attuned to the type of food we eat and meal timings, as well as how much we move around and the volume of water we drink. The gut even knows whether it is day or night and what time we usually go to the loo. If everything goes according to clockwork, the plan will be executed, and your bowels evacuated on schedule. Any disruption, such as altered sleep habits, travel or drastic dietary changes, will confuse the gut, which in turn affects your number two routine

---

Save yourself

Learning to take the strain out of your poo routine will cut down on the risk of haemorrhoids. It also vastly reduces the risk of a horror show called rectal prolapse. Basically, you bum isn't designed to telescope out of its housing. It's treatable, but painful and wholly avoidable. To save yourself the agony, aim to limit your time on the loo for number twos to a maximum of ten minutes, but ideally no more than five if you can manage it.

Also be sure to stay hydrated and aim to add about 30 grams of fibre to your daily diet. The fact is your faeces consist of water (about 75 per cent), bacteria and undigested fibre and it's the water and fibre in our diet that helps to keep stools soft, so they pass with the minimum of effort. It's not hard to achieve this intake in your diet: one apple, a handful of nuts and half a tin of beans will meet your daily fibre requirements, along with 6 to 8 cups of fluid.

Poo dynamics

Researchers have identified that homo sapiens can unleash faeces at a rate of up to 0.8 inches (about 2cm) per second, with the passage of an unobstructed stool taking on average 12 seconds. This figure is eerily consistent across most mammalian species, regardless of size.

This was the inspiration for an unusual but nonetheless interesting study performed in 2003 by Dov Sikirov, an Israeli physician who published his results in the journal *Digestive Diseases and Sciences*. He split his patients into three groups, each adopting different pooing positions. One group perched on a toilet that was 16 inches above ground, another settled on a 12-inch model, while the final group squatted and hovered over a plastic box on the ground.

He asked the participants to self-rate the ease of their bowel motions on a scale ranging from effortless to difficult, as well as record the total defecation time. Those on the 16-inch toilet reported taking over two minutes in total. The group on the 12-inch thrones performed a little quicker but both were outgunned by the squatters who opened their bowels in an average of 51 seconds. Those who simply leaned back on their haunches were also more likely to rate the experience towards the effortless end of the scale.

If we take this study as grounds to prove that squatting is a more effective and comfortable means of pooing, what on earth are we doing installing ourselves on toilet thrones?

To break the shitting shackles imposed on you by modern seating arrangements, you need to shift your position. Imagine if you will that your bowels are a long hosepipe and you're about to water your garden plants. Any curves and kinks in this hose means it takes longer for the water to reach the exit. The pressure will be dampened due to resistance. However, with a straightened hose, and with minimal resistance, the pressure and flow will be exquisite.

When you sit in your upright position to defecate, with your legs at 90-degree angles, you have to strain to navigate your faeces around a kink in the rectum created by the puborectalis, a pelvic floor muscle which forms a sling around your rectum. When you are standing upright, or even sitting down, this sling-like provides a welcome kink in your rectum to provide you with continence; the flow is disrupted. However, when you squat, this kink imposed by the puborectalis begins to unfurl and you have a clear run down the Hershey highway. If you chase the etymology of the word rectum, it even comes from the Latin 'rectus' which means straight. What's more, the act of squatting or simply bringing the knees up higher causes a rise in intrabdominal pressure and limits your need to strain.

Save yourself

So, how do we ensure a straight shot? Essentially there is an art to pooing for optimal efficiency and good health, and it's all about the angles.

First and foremost, a right angle is wrong. If the torso is at 90 degrees to the hips, the puborectalis muscle which hugs the rectum is in fact pulling extra tightly. This causes a kink in the tailpipe, compromising your optimum poo delivery as you don't have a clear drop down the rectum.

Next, adopt the squat. We're talking about the torso being at 35–60 degrees to the hips, which is effectively a squatting position or just try to get your knees higher than your hips. This can be easily achieved by sitting on the toilet with your feet resting on a stool (not that kind) or by leaning forwards whilst resting on the balls of your feet. It means the hips are relaxed and the puborectalis slackened. With the pinch point removed, you're free to poo without stresses or strains.

The canary in the coal mine

From soothsayers and mystics of the ancient world – who analysed animal droppings to glean some future prophesy – to doctors who obsessively pour over the minutiae of their patient's bowel motion, faecal matter has always maintained some link with health – and for good reason. Your bowel pattern and any significant changes to it can signal a deeper disturbance.

Once you've done the deed, it's always worth peering into the toilet after you poo. It might be grimly fascinating but more importantly it could save your life. The natural colour of human faeces ranges from brown to yellowish-brown. This is a healthy sign. Occasionally, it can change if something goes wrong, which is why keeping an eye on your poo can provide a useful insight into the goings-on of your gut.

If your poo is clay-coloured it suggests a lack of bile. This can mean there is a blockage in the pipes between the liver and the gut. Blocked passages in the body are never a good thing, and so those who notice any kind of grey-whiteish discoloration in their poo should consult a doctor.

Dark red or black faeces, known as malena, indicates the possibility of a bleeding point somewhere in the digestive tract. It also has an iron-like smell. Fresh blood is bright red and suggests either a major active bleed that is travelling so quickly through the intestine it has no time to be digested, or simply that it is somewhere beyond the stomach and small intestines (where most digestion occurs). Often the source of the bleed lies in the colon or anal region, possibly from a polyp or growth or something more benign like a haemorrhoid or a tear in the anal tissue – known as a fissure.

Beyond colour, a change in consistency is also a notable feature that can be linked to internal health. Persistent diarrhoea lasting for weeks can raise suspicion for intestinal inflammation, bowel cancer and even conditions affecting seemingly far removed organs like the thyroid (which can speed up gut motility if overactive). Stools that float and appear greasy could suggest a high fat content because your pancreas has been pummelled by infection, inflammation or alcohol and has shut down its production of the lipase enzyme that digests fat. Constipation, particularly that persists for several weeks and is a change from your usual routine, could be a warning sign of bowel cancer.

I should stress that constipation can also be a symptom of a range of health issues such as not drinking enough fluid or eating enough fibre to hormonal disturbances and diabetes. Constipation is rarely a diagnosis in its own right, merely a symptom of something else. Whatever the state of your shits, it can tell you a great deal about your state of health. Thankfully, there's no need for us to poke a finger in it. A universally recognised pictorial diagram called the Bristol Stool Chart helps us work out what's going on.

Rabbit-like pellets places you on a 2 or 3 and means you're probably constipated. In the first instance, this means you could benefit from an improved hydration routine and more fibre in your diet. If your turds score a healthy three or four on the scale then you have been blessed by the poo gods. Should your excrement look like it's been through a food

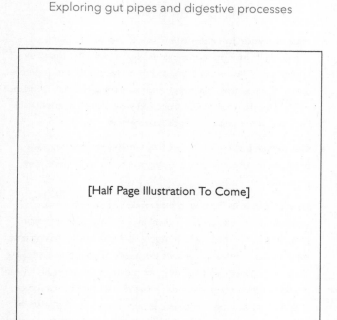

[Half Page Illustration To Come]

blender rather than your digestive tract, and needling into a 5, 6 or 7 on the scale, then chances are you've been beset by the diarrhoea demon.

Save yourself

Digestion problems can be uncomfortable at best. At worst, your body can use a poor diet and toilet routine to create enough problems to kill you, so, it's worth making friends with your intestines. A healthy relationship with your guts means your poo won't become a problem. As well as staying hydrated and not dodging the fruit, nuts, pasta and wholemeal bread for that all important fibre, here's how to keep your bowels in good shape:

- **Max out your microbiome** Think of the multitudinous organisms in your gut as live-in pets. If you look after them, they'll reward you. This means eating a wide range of foods to promote a diverse microbiome. Make sure your diet consists of an abundance of plant foods, wholegrains, fruits and vegetables that are high in fibre, and don't poo poo those polyphenols.

- **Get active** Building exercise into your daily routine is known to promote gut stimulation, helping you to move in more ways than one.

- **Don't hold it in** Prolonged suppression of defecation can significantly slow down your bowel movements. A little forward planning can help here, which largely comes down to making time for a regular toilet visit that suits the needs of your bowel's body clock. When it comes to pooing, what exactly does 'regular' mean? Frankly, there is no gold standard here. Everyone has a bespoke 'colonic transit time'. Some people poo three times a day while others have streamlined the process to three or four times a week. Your body knows best here, and if you can work with your bowels it'll improve efficiency when it comes to toilet visits.

- **Be consistent** Sticking to a toilet schedule, day in and day out, builds consistency in your bowel routine. The ideal time to go is after breakfast as this helps you tap into the gastrocolic reflex — when your stomach gives the green light to the intestines so they can start contracting. Just don't linger for more than a few minutes and avoid straining at all costs.

- **Be kind** The skin around your anus is thin and delicate. Harsh wiping can lead to tears in the rectum lining (anal fissures), which can lead to pain and bleeding. Wet wipes might seem like a good option, but they contain chemicals that can kill good bum bacteria. This can leave your back passage prone to bacterial, fungal and yeast infections. Wiping with dry toilet paper is OK, as long as you do so from front to back to avoid the genital area (a case in point for women in particular), but really not much different than using dry leaves. Ultimately, water is the way forward. A bidet – like a toilet with an upward-facing tap – is the best way to wash your anus, but if you're not posh enough to own one than dampening the toilet paper will do. Just be sure to pat dry before resuming your day.

A final word on gut instincts

We know an information superhighway exists between the gastrointestinal system and the brain and that it's critical to our physical and mental health. But have you ever had a 'gut feeling?', an instinct that seemed low on evidence but irrefutable? Did you ever wonder why that was?

Your gut instinct or intuition is not philosophy; it's science. It is an interplay between your brain and gut, with both working in tandem to synthesise data from your past decisions, experiences, memories and excess information you don't perceive in your conscious state. Ultimately this provides you with a nebulous feeling that seems emotional yet congruent. Although it may feel guttural, visceral and a case of emotions over facts, these subconscious cues are rooted in biology.

A gut feeling has been the inspiration for works of art, the winning ingredient for many a professional athlete and the first step towards discovering that your partner is living a double life. In some cultures, this weird sixth sense has even been interpreted as something divined from the gods, like a supernatural gift of foresight. In real terms, it's a complex series of neurotransmitter signals and electric sparks courtesy of the enteric nervous system; a name for the mesh of neurons embedded within the GI system.

Short of being more sentient than you, the latest research even suggests that your gut microbes help make decisions about what foods they want and thus what you crave. Having perused the metaphorical menu, these hungry bugs can send chemical signals to your brain nudging you to consume whatever they need for their own survival. *Waiter*!

Regardless of how we make sense of it in our lives, our understanding of the gut–brain interaction will prove pivotal for the future of medicine. Ultimately, it represents potential for major breakthroughs regarding how certain diseases appear to formulate in the gut before making their way to our next subject under the operating theatre lights: the brain.

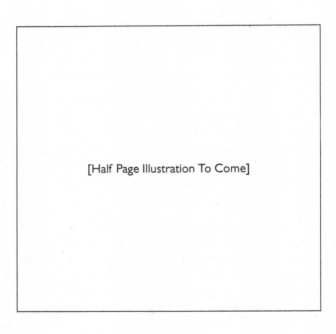

[Half Page Illustration To Come]

Health Hack

If you're prescribed antibiotics, which don't just nuke the bad bacteria but also the good guys, here's a simple way to minimise the inevitable digestive disruption:

* Increase your fibre intake (nuts, seeds, vegetables and beans) to encourage good bacteria to thrive.

* Alternatively, consider a fibre supplement such as psyllium husk (available from health food shops). This is commonly available as a soluble mix that's gentle on the gut.

2. The Lights Are On . . .

ALL ABOUT THE BRAIN

IN SOFTWARE TERMS, your brain is comparable to an early computer operating system. It's riddled with bad code, slow to load when you need it most, and plays to all the wrong strengths. This so-called state-of-the-art processor enjoys watching cat memes more than going to sleep, despite one such activity being demonstrably better for it than the other. Looking at the brain's various glitches and flaws, you'd be forgiven for thinking it was constructed by a team of failed engineers with a drinking problem.

An unappetising chunk of flesh in a bony cage, your brain weighs around 1.3kg. Despite amounting to no more than 2 per cent of your body weight, it is huge drain on your natural resources. On average, your brain consumes 20 per cent of your energy reserves.

Setting aside performance issues, your brain is a surprisingly intricate structure, containing somewhere in the ballpark of a 100 billion neurons. These are cells that form your body's information highway. They communicate with each other through eco-friendly electrical and chemical signals. Each zap jumps across tiny gaps between the neurons called synapses. In a flash, they can shuttle information all the way from your brain to your index finger, just so you can pick your nose.

The human brain isn't satisfied with managing eating, breathing and pooing. Today, it wants to get complicated and try its hand at art, poetry and getting TikTok memes off the ground. The problem is that the operating system housed in your skull wasn't designed to do many of the things we surround ourselves with in modern life. To be honest, we're crying out for a new system to drop. Until that happens, here we are. Like all of us, you'll just have to keep on stumbling through life and hope that the central control unit keeps pulling all the right strings.

The organ that named itself

The first time I held a human brain in my hands, it was a lot heavier than I expected. Don't worry, I wasn't in the basement wearing my beloved leather mask. This was during an anatomy session in my first year at medical school.

As the course progressed, the anatomy tutor presented various brains to us, some already sliced open to reveal the cross-sectional anatomy. The brain is filled with various lobes, as well as chambers known as ventricles, and has an intricate pattern of nerve fibres and grooves known as fissures. Every time I was presented with one, I thought to myself that this delicate blob once supported someone's hopes, dreams and emotions. It burned brightly throughout an entire life, but now that light was off.

Many years after my first hands-on experience with a brain, I assisted in a neurosurgical case. Here, I discovered that a *live* human brain has a consistency more akin to cottage cheese than a cadaveric specimen. Dead brains feel more like a cold, slippery cauliflower, especially when heavy with preservation chemicals. (Please don't read this bit out loud in public.)

The human brain looks like a walnut (which, as it happens, is a particularly good 'brain food'), although it is in fact separated into halves. These are joined together by a bundle of nerve fibres known as the corpus callosum. While some brain functions are split between each half – for example the left side of your body is largely controlled by the right side of your brain and vice versa – the two brain hemispheres do not operate independently as many wrongly claim. You might have heard someone say they are 'right-brained' or 'left-brained', suggesting that one particular hemisphere is dominant. This stems from the idea that the left side handles more creative functions while the right side shines at organisational or analytical skills. It may be true that certain brain regions seem to specialise at specific tasks like visual or language processing. However, there is currently no hard science to evidence that anyone has one dominant brain half or possesses a personality determined in this way. You're not that special.

The two halves of the brain are in constant communication. They also produce results in tandem. In fact, almost every action you take is distributed across multiple regions of your entire brain. Thanks to eerie, split-brain experiments in which a patient's corpus callosum is severed (an old-fashioned treatment for severe epilepsy) and by studying stroke patients, we have gained a solid understanding of the differences between the two brain halves.

Unfortunately, when it comes to brain matters, nothing is as simple as it first appears. The idea of split brain function is almost as preposterous as the myth that you only use 10 per cent of your brain. To put it simply, you use 100 per cent of your brain for various things all the time. There isn't any hidden unlocked potential we are suppressing. Yours is as good as it gets.

Even though it's constantly firing on all cylinders, the brain can still surprise us. What if I told you that there are documented cases of people incurring brain injuries that actually resulted in them becoming *smarter*. Some have even acquired the capabilities of a genius. Or stranger yet, there was a person who lived almost their entire life totally normally, essentially without a brain?

Setting aside my view that we could all do with a new model to thrive in the modern world, your brain is the most complex thing in the universe. It's also the most important organ in your body, according to your brain at any rate. Suspicious.

It is the organ that named itself, because without a brain we'd be without the power of thought, self-awareness and language. As a result, it has appointed itself as the nexus of our being. In theory, a full understanding of the brain would require a complete understanding of consciousness, and perhaps life, the universe and everything – though my bet is on that answer being forty-two, of course.

So, how do we study the brain? Unfortunately, neuroscience and neurology possess some unique challenges compared with other sciences. While brain scans and MRIs can showcase activity in a conscious person, it's very difficult to understand how this directly creates conscious experience or intelligence. It's certainly true that we can learn a lot from *dissecting* a brain. It's just not immediately obvious which areas of the brain are responsible for different functions when you do so.

Probably one of the most famous brains that has ever been dissected is that of Albert Einstein. Within seven and a half hours of his death, Einstein's brain was removed from his dead body and subsequently cut up into 240 blocks. In accordance with his last wishes, this was undertaken in the name of science (and, I suspect, to eliminate the possibility of a genius zombie rising from the dead). Examination of the samples showed that Einstein's brain did have some minor differences from other brains, such as a slightly denser corpus callosum: the area of the brain that connects the two cerebral hemispheres and allows for communication between them. Nevertheless, in the vast majority of ways it was the *same*.

So, if cutting up brains doesn't help us much, how can we effectively study them?

The answer: patients with brain damage. Some of the best data in neuroscience comes from looking at patients who survive brain injuries and examining how their personalities and lives change afterwards. This gives us an extraordinary before-and-after experiment that would be unethical to intentionally perform. It also brings us to the case of Phineas Gage, which sounds like it should be a Sherlock Holmes story, now that I think about it.

When brains go boom

Phineas Gage is neuroscience's most famous patient. He was born in the USA in 1823 and grew up to become a railroad construction foreman.

Then, at the age of twenty-five, an accident happened that would transform our understanding of the human brain.

Gage was working with demolition explosives to remove an outcrop of rock. Moments before he pushed the plunger, he was distracted by men working nearby. On turning, he accidentally moved into the line of the tamping iron. This long, heavy rod is used to plug explosive material into rock, and can shoot out like a rocket on detonation.

The result wasn't pretty. The tamping iron blasted up through the left side of Gage's face. Moving upwards, it passed through his lower jaw, behind his left eye, through the left side of the brain, and then exited the top of his skull through the frontal bone.

Almost unbelievably, Gage didn't die. In fact, he was conscious and speaking within *a few minutes of the accident*. He was even able to walk with some help. But the strangest part of the story happens after the accident. Not only did Gage survive the accident, but he also lived for another twelve years. It wasn't just a second chance at life; such was the profound change to his personality that some felt Gage to be a different person altogether.

Before the accident, Gage was considered to be hard-working, responsible, and a general standout guy. Afterwards, he became impulsive, uninhibited, and just plain old rude. The change was so stark that the people who knew him said he was 'no longer Gage'.

The main part of the brain that Gage lost was from his frontal lobe. This is an area of the brain associated with self-control and higher-level thinking. Despite the severity of his injuries, however, it was noted that Gage's memory and attention were still relatively intact.

To conclude this remarkable story, and with due credit to the determination of his family, Gage went on to regain his old social skills. For the rest of his life, he returned to his former self, despite missing a large chunk of his brain. While he died from an epileptic seizure, which was no doubt associated with the accident, Gage's extraordinary survival provided critical insight into brain function. In summary, like a relationship break-up, it's complicated.

Why bother with a brain?

Odd stories like the Gage case illustrate not only how much we now know about the brain, but also how much we've yet to truly understand. Essentially, our brains must continue to study themselves, and maybe one day we can find a way to make us all on a par with Einstein. In the meantime, though, it's a good idea to avoid brain injury as far as possible. A meta-analysis performed by the *European Journal of Neurology* shows that almost all impairments are purely negative. So, if you're cramming for an exam, it's not a good idea to ask your mate to launch a golf ball at your head.

Saturday night in the emergency room

Sadly, the majority of head injuries will not improve your life. During my time working in emergency rooms, I have come across many a patient presenting a problem relating to their brain. All too often, when they arrived dazed and bleeding, it's clearly injury-related, from assault, a fall or a road traffic accident. Then there are those who come in with a severe headache. I always hope it's down to a migraine, which can be debilitating, but sometimes it can be the symptom of an insidious tumour.

Anyone that has ever worked in an emergency room knows that weekends are notorious for bringing in late-night revellers with all manner of drunken injuries and overdoses. One such time, I was manning the 'resus' bay with my senior. This is where trauma patients will come first to be stabilised. So, when the paramedics brought in a young man who had been assaulted outside a nightclub, he was delivered into our care.

The young man was only slightly lucid. His eyes remained closed and mostly he just moaned in response to questions. He complained of a severe headache and nausea, and was clearly confused as he believed he was still in the nightclub. The paramedics said they had found him unconscious at the scene. Having examined him briefly, my instincts told me this was worse than it seemed. His left pupil was fixed and dilated; this is never a good sign and usually suggests a significant brain injury. His breathing was slightly irregular, his pulse low at 55 beats per minutes and his blood pressure higher than expected for a young man, sitting at 180/80; again not good. These were also signs of something we learn about in medical school but very rarely see in clinical practice: Cushing's triad. This is a physiological response to rising intracranial pressure, suggesting, in this case, a bleed in the brain.

I ordered a CT scan, which was carried out with urgency. On the screen, my attention focused on a lemon-shaped mass in one quarter of the skull. This characteristic shape develops due to a rapidly expanding mass of blood called a haematoma. In this instance, it was stuck between the skull and the dura – the membrane covering the brain – which literally translates from Latin as 'hard mother'.

This type of bleed is known as an extradural haematoma. It can compress the brain because of the increasing pressures of the collecting blood. Eventually, with enough pressure in the skull, parts of the brain can be squeezed out of the skull; this is known as herniation and can lead to death. As a result, the patient was transferred to a special neurosurgical unit for treatment as a matter of urgency. In cases like this, effective treatment depends on speed. It can't be rushed, but equally there is no time for hesitation or delay. It's only afterwards, when the diagnosis has been made and the patient is receiving appropriate care, that I can pause to reflect. Any incident like this just underlines both the wonder, complexity and fragility of the brain, and how central it is to our lives. It might sound obvious, and yet sometimes we need to be reminded because it operates out of sight and (you might say) mind. While my role in that young man's care had come to an end, I hope he made a full recovery.

The culprit in 75 per cent of these types of brain bleeds is in a region known as the pterion: the weakest part of the skull. It's an area where four different skull bones fuse together and is particularly vulnerable to injury as the bone is very thin. Directly underneath the pterion is the middle meningeal artery. With little bone to protect it, this is an artery that can be easily ruptured. This vulnerable area aside, the skull is fairly handy; it's basically the inbuilt human version of a crash helmet for the brain. It's not a perfect design by any means, otherwise there would be no need to build actual crash helmets to protect your noggin.

Punch drunk

Head injuries don't just have to be one-off, violent or involve bleeding to cause issues. Many low-grade head injuries, while seemingly innocuous, can prove over time to be just as sinister and destructive.

The list of former boxers who have demonstrated declining cognitive abilities after retirement, from severe memory loss to poor coordination and often personality changes, is exhaustive. This syndrome is often referred to as dementia pugilistica (boxer's dementia or fighter's dementia). We now use the term CTE, or chronic traumatic encephalopathy, which is defined as a progressive neurodegenerative disease associated with repetitive traumatic brain injuries. It isn't just seen in boxing but also in virtually every contact sport, from rugby to American football.

Contact sports that involve repeated, low- to moderate-impact head trauma all carry a risk of causing concussion, which is considered to be a mild brain injury. It can result from being struck on the head by anything from a ball, a bat or another player.

The word 'concussion' is derived from concutere, which is Latin for 'to shake violently' and this is exactly what happens inside your skull. The brain is serenely floating in its protective bath of cerebrospinal fluid only to be knocked like a pinball against the skull. The force required to do this is surprisingly minimal. It isn't always associated with a knockout, but it can cause neuronal damage.

Over time, a person who has suffered from just one concussion like this can find themselves at increased risk of dementia. In fact, one of the largest studies looking at the impact of head trauma on the brain involving, 15,000 participants (the PROTECT study), found that three or more concussions had a significantly more deleterious effect on a person's cognitive function, which exponentially worsened with each subsequent concussion. In simple terms, more brain bashing is bad.

This is believed to be associated with changes to the brain 'washing' process that naturally occurs in the skull. Here – and generally when you're asleep – cerebrospinal fluid washes over your brain to give it a bath. This clears toxic waste products and debris that fill up during the day, and it's believed that traumatic head injuries can interfere with this process. It can impact on quality of sleep, and has been linked to an increased risk of neurodegenerative conditions.

If there's anything to take away from all this it's a simple lesson: protect your head like you would your nether regions. After all, you don't tolerate low- to moderate-grade impacts to your genitals every day.

HACKING THE BRAIN

Like any outdated computer operating system, your brain is prone to vulnerabilities. Bugs and viruses are constantly knocking on its doors. This can be bad news, of course, but not always. The system is also quite easy to hack; again, this could be catastrophic, but in the hands of good guys (i.e. you) it's possible to tweak the brain and enhance performance. Let's look at the main players in turn.

Eat yourself smarter

Right now, it's highly likely that your brain is under the control of hundreds of microscopic pathogenic puppet masters. (I've introduced you to these little guys before.) We know gut microbes do more than assist in digestion and metabolism of what we eat; they also help synthesise certain neurotransmitters, in the form of chemicals like dopamine and serotonin, which have important roles to play in your central nervous system. In fact, these gut bugs have a direct red-carpet route to your brain via the vagus nerve, which has receptors adjacent to the gut lining. This host–microbe interplay is a very dynamic one and is far from a one-way street; the brain state can equally have an effect on the lives of gut flora. Stress, for example, can increase inflammation, thus disrupting the gut landscape and the population of bacterial species.

Save yourself

If your gut microbes are unhappy, their mood can manifest itself in a number of ways in your brain, from bringing you down to brain fog and beyond. A chronically poor diet heavy in processed foods can also lead to a build-up of cholesterol in the arteries. This can impact on blood flow to the brain thus affecting its function. Make your diet heathy and balanced and it won't just be your gut that thanks you but also your brain.

To provide the brain with blood, as well as oxygen and nutrients, you need iron to do the heavy lifting and transportation logistics. It's also needed by the enzymes that produce neurotransmitters. Low iron levels can result in anaemia, which can manifest with symptoms like fatigue, lethargy and low concentration and mood.

Vitamin D is another key supplement that regulates mood. Magically (and some might go so far as to say dark arts must be involved) the body manufactures most of its supply from sunshine. Traditionally, it's a vitamin associated with bone and muscle health, but in truth its remit extends much further than that. This steroid hormone (it's not technically a vitamin) is also involved in memory function and a deficiency of vitamin D can cause low mood, which is why people sometimes suffer from seasonal affective disorder in the winter months when sunshine is in limited supply.

Mood regulation also relies heavily on adequate protein intake (found in poultry, seafood, pasta, dairy, nuts, beans and eggs to name a few). It's crucial in the synthesis of the neurotransmitters serotonin and dopamine, both of which regulate mood.

Neurotransmitters and hormones are one thing but for the brain cells to respond to them adequately you need decent levels of zinc (found in wholegrains, nuts and breakfast cereals).

One of the most important elements required in a diet is omega-3. These fatty acids are involved in building the brain's cell membranes and there are three types: eicosapentaenoic acid (EPA), docosahexaenoic acid (DHA) and alpha-linoleic acid (ALA). The first two are found in oily fish like salmon and the latter is found in leafy greens and nuts (spinach and walnuts). While the body can convert ALA to EPA/DHA, the best way to get EPA and DHA is through the consumption of fish. It's worth noting that omega-3 supplements haven't yet shown the same effects as the omega-3 found in food sources.

In the fog

When it comes to the pathogenic effects on the brain by microscopic marauders like viruses, we only have to look at the current cases of long Covid, also known as 'Covid Brain'. It's a seemingly insidious and long-lasting hangover from even a mild case of the Covid-19 virus. Even though no longer testing positive for the virus, sufferers report memory loss, lack of motivation and focus and low mood, and this can last for weeks, months and sometimes longer. Additionally, scientists have noticed significant structural changes to the brain (as seen on MRI scans) both before and after infection. In some instances, the brain of a patient with long Covid has shrunk in size with a decreased density of grey matter in regions associated with memory.

Throughout the pandemic, healthcare professionals the world over documented that the Covid virus didn't simply attack the lungs but even distant body parts like the brain. They noted neurological symptoms in their patients and evidence of encephalopathy (a general term for injury to the brain).

Research into long Covid is still in its infancy, but the number of cases cannot be ignored. There's no doubt that it's the post viral condition of our times, but a glance back through history shows that our brains have been collateral damage in the wake of previous pandemics.

One of the most infamous cases was the strange worldwide phenomenon of extreme fatigue and exhaustion which plagued millions of people soon after the 1918 influenza outbreak. This post-viral syndrome was dubbed 'sleepy sickness' or encephalitis lethargica. It was believed that the influenza virus impacted on the dopamine-producing neurons of the central nervous system. More than simply experiencing fatigue, patients were crippled by severe clinical depression and apathy. There is perhaps a lesson to be learned here for our response to future viral pandemics. Fighting the initial fire is one thing, but what's left in the debris can be equally damaging.

It's not a medical or scientific term, but 'brain fog' accurately captures the sense of mental slowing and disorientation that many patients feel when they experience cognitive impairment after chronic fatigue syndrome, a brain injury or a post-viral illnesses. Even women in the midst of menopause are known to suffer from this disruptive state of mind. If you've ever felt like you can't concentrate or focus well, or simply struggle to remember stuff that would otherwise come to you in a flash, then it's likely that you have experienced a degree of brain fog. It's not uncommon, even if it often goes unreported as people often just try to press on through it.

Brain fog can also be triggered and exacerbated by non-physical causes too; namely emotional and social stressors. For example, since 2020 a huge number of people not infected by Covid-19 have also experienced extreme tiredness and other cognitive issues. Research is ongoing, with attention focused on pandemic stress, lockdowns and working from home.

'Have you turned it on and off again?'

The brain is like one of those frustrating old operating systems. Chances are you've grown to depend on it. More often than not it makes life easy for you. Sometimes, it's capable of producing moments of genius; occasionally, however, it reveals itself as nothing more than a blob of inefficient jelly. Despite its shortcomings, you've grown to live with it just fine. So, let's look at some of its weird characteristics and the workarounds you've subconsciously crafted to stay functioning.

• Access restrictions

Often, your brain doesn't have the right credentials and security clearance to influence certain bodily functions. Even if it thinks that it does have the authority, your organs sometimes ignore it. Your brain has never issued a direct instruction to store fat. Neither has it ordered you to feel aroused during a business meeting or funeral service. But it happens.

Even when it does call the shots, your brain often only has a flimsy, indirect control of certain functions. This is enabled through automatic default pathways called reflexes, which are often poorly suited for purpose. An example is goosebumps, also known as the pilomotor reflex. This occurs when the arrector pilae muscle at the base of a hair follicle contracts and causes the skin to form a bump. It's useful for our feathered or furry predecessors to help them warm up but is useless for us. Unless we believe in ghosts.

Our brain has no root privileges for our body. It can't log on to admin or switch into developer mode. We are simply a vessel to contain genes, which in fact are the true executive board.

Then there's the issue of maintenance. For optimal performance, the brain has to switch into sleep mode for up to eight hours and sometimes longer on a daily basis. It's a vital function, and yet the setting is frequently corrupted by unintelligible information in the form of dreams and nightmares.

• Storage space and corrupt files

Sitting through hours upon hours of often useless lectures at medical school (at least it seemed that way at the time), I usually felt my brain was brimming with information to the point it felt 'full'. Even though I often feel that I couldn't process any more information, our capacity for storage is something software giants would kill to replicate. No matter how overloaded we can sometimes feel, we never have to worry about running low on disk space in our lifetimes.

We have approximately one billion neurons in our brain. With each neuron forming 1,000 connections to other neurons, that amounts to more than one trillion connections, so you might be forgiven for thinking this means we have a trillion data points worth of memory. In reality, each neuron involves itself with more than just one memory, thus exponentially increasing your storage capacity.

All these comparisons between our brain's memory capacity and computer storage should be taken with a pinch of salt. We still don't know what it takes to store a singular memory. In fact, we've no idea what a singular memory consists of. Just know you have ample space.

For all its storage potential, the fact remains that as a processing unit our brain is a mess. The hard drive becomes saturated with junk information and the useful data becomes increasingly difficult to access with ease. Add to this a recall function that slows with age, corrupted memory files and random crucial data that gets deleted when we need it the most, not to mention disease and the general proclivity of our memory filing cabinets to falsify memory documents, and you have a heady storm of sloppy administration.

• False memories

I hope you're sitting down for this. Your memories are mostly made up. They're a fiction. You brain doesn't record memories like a video. Instead, it takes snapshots of the most important elements. Then, when you recall the event, the brain just guesses what happened in between each snapshot, based on past experience and a heft dollop of generalisation. This is why it's easy to implant false memories in ourselves or convince someone else that a false memory is a true; this is evidenced by numerous legal cases in which suspects recalled 'false memories' under duress of interrogation.

In fact, just by thinking about the past, you're erasing your memory. Each time you think about a memory you're not actually recalling the actual event; you're simply thinking about the last time you thought about that memory. What this means is that each time you recall something you're actually creating a copy of that memory, which is less accurate than the one before that, and the one before that, and so on. Your memory recall is basically a long running game of telephone.

BECOMING BRAIN EFFICIENT

When you make demands on your computer, usually by loading up some processor-hungry game, it can cause the fan to kick in to stop it from overheating. The brain doesn't possess that kind of fail-safe, but it can make mistakes if you're asking too much of it.

When I'm watching TV, for example, I have to remind myself to stop scrolling through social media on my phone. Multitasking erodes your productivity and task efficiency. It results in an increased error rate and higher levels of inaccuracies. Often, this obliges you to perform the tasks again but separately, so you are essentially becoming less productive. Whatever way you spin it, constant task-switching reduces the quality and efficiency of your work. In fact, one limited study from the University of Sussex looked at the MRI scans of individuals who multitasked (texted and watched TV). It found a reduced density in the anterior cingulate cortex, an area of the brain involved in empathy and emotional regulation.

What's more, your constant shifting attention from one thing to another results in the prefrontal cortex and striatum burning rapidly through oxygenated glucose. This can leave you feeling exhausted after even short bursts of multitasking because you've literally depleted your brain's energy reserves. Yes, it's commendable that you've tried to do everything at once. In reality, your brain's just fried and you've accidentally sent a private pic to the group chat.

Background music benefits

There is no doubt your brain performs at its best when focusing on one thing at a time. Even so, you can make an exception when it comes to listening to music while you work. We have two attention systems: a conscious and an unconscious one. When you're deeply focused on a piece of work your unconscious attention can be distracted by the sound effects of life: phone notifications or creaks in the floor can divert the focus from your conscious attention. A low-key input like an ambient soundtrack can act as a buffer, however, and suppress these noises to keep our unconscious attention busy. It's like giving a dog a bone to play with while you get on with the important stuff.

Rhythmic thinking

There is one more great efficiency saving for your brain. It comes to down to getting in tune with your natural body clock. Humans are bound by several cycles, but the one under the spotlight here is known as the ultradian rhythm, and falling into step with it can only benefit your brain.

The ultradian rhythm is a repeated biological cycle that takes place in 90-minute waves within a 24-hour cycle. Ultradian literally means 'many times a day'. It has a role to play in managing energy production and recovery and isn't just limited to humans. Plants, animals, fungi and various other living things are bound by it too.

When you're asleep these ultradian cycles are involved in your REM (rapid eye movement) patterns. During the day, however, they're crucial in influencing your performance and energy levels. In the first part of what is a roughly 90-minute cycle, physiological parameters like your heart rate, brain activity, hormone levels and alertness all rise. Approaching the end of that cycle, they subsequently decline. In other words, we perform best when we focus on intense work for up to 90 minutes, followed by a 20-minute break. By following this rough ultradian cycle, you can effectively optimise your performance to closely match the natural ebb and flow of body.

EXTENDING THE WARRANTY

The ravages of time will eventually claim your brain. Early in life, it's literally a sponge for knowledge. After the first twenty years, however, it becomes harder to retain new information. This is down to a steady cognitive decline. The good news is it can be slowed. Like a well-cared for machine, there are many ways to fine-tune it to ensure optimal performance for longer.

Switch on

Automation has made us less reliant on our natural cognitive resources for basic tasks like simple arithmetic. We use our car's navigation systems for the same routes we use every day. We might even drive off in a vehicle that changes gear for us automatically. Eventually these things become crutches we rely on, and that eats away at our brain function. To counter this, make sure you still continue to test your brain every now and then.

It isn't just a question of switching off the satnav. Learning a new skill or language will encourage your brain to stretch itself. For example, getting to grips with a musical instrument calls into play your memory, motor coordination skills, attention and hearing skills. There is even research to suggest musicians are less inclined to develop dementia than those who don't play any instruments. Similar evidence is available for speaking more than one language. *C'est simple, non?*

Get ahead

As well as maintaining a healthy diet and staying hydrated, exercise is one of the most effective ways to fortify your mind. It doesn't simply improve body-wide blood flow, which extends to the brain, but also stimulates various nerve growth factors than can sustain and maintain neural pathways. Although this thing that sits between our ears isn't really a muscle, one of the revelations in the field of neuroscience in the last couple of decades is that the brain does seem to function like one. It's plastic and malleable and with practice, it changes dynamically in response to what you do; if left alone it can atrophy. One thing we know with absolute certainty is that aerobic exercise such as walking or running can materially increase the volume of the hippocampus, a brain region associated with memory. Even more amazing is that this neuroplasticity of the brain is retained throughout life; so an old dog can learn new tricks simply by building in a regular exercise routine.

Find your tribe

Humans are social creatures. So, it makes sense that isolation can have profoundly negative effects on our brain and mental health. Furthermore, there is evidence to suggest that increasing contact with friends and family – and generally enjoying social activities – helps to stave off cognitive decline. Social interactions don't just boost mood but higher cognitive abilities such as memory, attention and focus.

Rebel against retirement

A number of studies associate retirement with cognitive decline. There are numerous reasons for this, but ultimately we know that mental and social stimulation are key players. When you remove these factors, health deteriorates. Keeping mentally active raises something known as your 'cognitive reserve'. This is your brain's ability to fight off the cognitive effects of ageing. When that core social network is removed, health declines.

We've learned that staying active, social and stimulated is key to keeping your brain in shape. It means we need to stop looking at retirement as a time to unwind and instead consider it to be an opportunity to expand our horizons. That comfy armchair you've had your eye on for the last twenty-five years? Mark my words, the moment you put your feet up is when the rot can set into both your mind and body. Keep stimulated and you stand a good chance of remembering your own name for some time to come.

Relax

One of the greatest emotions that overcomes me during busy shifts and difficult surgeries is stress. I used to underestimate just how pronounced its effects can be on the body and specifically the mind. When you experience stress, your brain flips a switch that results in a cascade of hormones – cortisol, adrenaline and noradrenaline, the so-called stress hormones – which activate the 'fight or flight response'.

In the short term, washing your brain with these chemicals can be very useful. It can aid people in coping with a threat or danger, help an athlete run faster or a tired surgeon operate with more dexterity and intensity. However, your brain can't handle too much of a good thing. It's fussy, and can only manage a specific degree of stress. Too much, or a prolonged elevation of stress hormones, can cause a stressful event to spill into generalised anxiety. Chronic elevation of stress chemicals like cortisol can also affect the prefrontal cortex, a brain region involved in emotional processing, executive decision making (planning, problem-solving) and attention.

Stress is a vicious cycle. Not only can it affect and shrink the rational prefrontal cortex, but it can also increase the size of the brain's fear centre, the amygdala. In turn, this makes the brain even more susceptible to stress. In essence, these stress chemicals create a domino effect. When tipped, they reinforce neural pathways in the brain so a person is more prone to being in a constant state of anxiety.

In my first year as a doctor on a busy respiratory ward in peak winter, the late hours, busy shifts and lack of self-care eventually took their toll. For me, this resulted in insomnia and the occasional bout of palpitations.

To remedy this, I aimed to shape up my sleep routine to improve the quality of my shut-eye. I also got into a regular exercise routine, which helped me enormously. These small changes to my life helped to reduce the deleterious effects of stress on the brain, namely inflammation.

As well the holistic improvements, I also wanted instant fixes I could call upon in those moments when my stress levels needled. Working in a hospital, I found that stressful situations could come thick and fast, from encounters with angry patients to disagreements with colleagues or frustrations with lagging IT systems. I found deep-breathing exercises a particularly effective way to bring my heart rate down and call off the panic klaxon in my brain. This wasn't just effective in countering big stresses, I discovered, but crucially the more common micro-stresses that accumulate throughout the day and eventually tip you over the edge.

Good sleep, regular exercise and an annoying tendency to come over all zen on my colleagues worked wonders in keeping my stress in check. The most effective technique of all, I found, was in learning to channel my inner dolphin.

Yes, it sounds like a euphemism that could get me struck off and lose my license. In reality, it is one of the most effective, science-based, stress-busting brain resets I can employ.

Every one of us is hard-wired with an archaic feature called the mammalian diving reflex. This is triggered when you plunge your face into cold water while holding your breath. If you don't fancy this, splashing your face and nostrils also works (just not as well!). Once the face is underwater and your nostrils full of water, this information is relayed to the brain by the trigeminal nerve (fifth cranial nerve). In turn, this pushes the vagus nerve (tenth cranial nerve) to induce bradycardia, also known as a lowering of the heart rate. This prompts the blood vessels to narrow, which restricts flow into the limbs to preserve it for the heart, brain and lungs. The combination of these physiological changes is known to decrease anxiety and stress. So, next time you're finding it hard to cope, find a restorative source of cold water.

THE PAIN GAME

We are continually uncovering interesting things about the brain, and yet it still hasn't fully revealed itself to us. Despite our apparent advances, the fact is we aren't that far from knowing what our ancestors understood. It's an enigmatic organ.

Back then (I mean way back then to the tune of 8,000 years ago), the oldest surgical procedure was born. In short, it involved creating a hole in someone's skull. The act of trepanation, as it's called, was considered to be a solution to all kinds of physical and mental health problems. It was the means by which our cave-dwelling ancestors sought to exorcise 'bad spirits', while our medieval cousins figured that breaking into the skull could cure severe headaches. Yes, death was no doubt quite an effective means of easing the pain, and quickly considered to be overkill. Surprisingly, we still employ the hole-in-the-head method in modern medicine. The only difference is that we do it with a slightly less ham-fisted approach than our forebears. Today, a craniotomy (as it has been rebranded) is predominantly used as an emergency manoeuvre by neurosurgeons to evacuate blood accumulation in the brain.

In their ivory towers of medicine, neurosurgeons have advanced their art to the point where they even perform brain surgery while patients are awake. This is possible because the brain has no pain receptors. In keeping a patient conscious, it means surgeons can constantly monitor basic responses to assess the effects of the procedure.

Understanding pain

Unlike the brain, which cannot perceive pain, everything around it will cry out at the slightest provocation. From the surrounding blood vessels to the membranous covering (the meninges), as well as the nerves and neck muscles, we're talking about sensitive flowers who like to cause a drama. It explains why a stiff neck or pain in the scalp can lead to tension headaches, while cold substances like ice cream give rise to 'brain freeze', aka sphenopalatine ganglioneuralgia.

But what exactly is pain? At its most basic level, it's a mechanism by which our brain provides us with an unpleasant sensation to try to stop or change our behaviour. Sometimes this goes wildly wrong or the switch is permanently flipped to 'on' mode in the form of chronic pain. This systemic glitch can prove deeply disruptive to the lives of sufferers, not to mention proving costly for society to manage.

I have frequently been involved in an operation to remove someone's entire colon, rectum and anus, typically if they suffer with inflammatory bowel disease. This procedure, called a pan-proctocolectomy, is often referred to very informally as Barbie butt surgery. This is because the anus is removed and stitched closed as part of the procedure. One not so rare side effect from this surgery can be something known as 'phantom rectum' syndrome, where patients still feel the urge to go to the toilet despite there being nothing there. Most cases of phantom limb might be explained by simple cross-wiring, or damaged nerves that recover but poorly and feed erroneous signals to the brain. In the case of the phantom rectum, it may be a damaged pudendal nerve still feeding false messages to the brain, resulting in the individual literally being haunted by ghost poos.

Nowadays, we have moved away from the naive model of thinking that pain is just a correlate of tissue damage. We now know you can suffer pain without injury. The issue remains, however, that we only really know how to treat it effectively when we identify not just where it hurts, but also why.

Name the pain

The majority of people will deal with pain in their lives. Some will experience it far more than others. I've always found that my patients were able to better cope with their pain once they understood the causes and possible treatments. In an odd way, pain education provides some indirect analgesic support.

Theatre of pain

Your paranoid brain is so overprotective it creates the sensation of pain from within itself. Like a hallucination, it can haunt your every waking moment. The science on this is crystal clear. While your tissue may relay signals to your brain, pain is in fact a proprietary product of Brain Inc. In other words, the receptors on your burned hand do not send pain signals to the brain. It just sends signals.

The sensory signals received from injured tissues are just one of the variables the brain assimilates to create its theatrical experience of pain. The pain you feel having foolishly bitten your inner cheek when gorging on your second chocolate bar of the evening isn't coming from the cheek. The sensation is combined with previous memories, cultural beliefs and other sensory data to produce an experience.

Sometimes when the mood takes it, this calculating mastermind exaggerates the pain signals; this is known as hyperalgesia. The brain can cry wolf one too many times, however. This results in sensitisation, in which you just put up with the apparent discomfort because you know that it'll pass.

Behind the drama, the truth is that your brain isn't great at deciphering the source of all pain. Often, it just makes a very well-educated guess based on incoming and previously stored data. Referred pain is a classic example. That backache you feel might actually be produced by your abdomen, which can cause diagnostic dilemmas.

Fine-tuning the 'pain signal'

Bombshell alert: biology class lied to you. There is no such thing as a pain signal or pain fibres that detect pain. Nociceptors (the so-called pain receptors) detect noxious stimuli which can cause pain; like the time you stepped on a piece of Lego at 4am while going to the bathroom. The noxious stimuli are interpreted by the brain, which then decides how to respond. So, when the sole of your foot closes over that spikey plastic brick one night, you might walk on without noticing or you might hit the ceiling with a curse.

The sensation and perception of pain is actually a two-way street. The brain can receive 'pain' signals but also feed them back to those sensory nerves to tune up or tune down pain in line with how it wants to perceive it. This may go some way to explain how fakirs, ascetics who have denounced worldly pleasures, can tolerate sitting on a bed of nails or Shaolin monks can take violent kicks to the crown jewels.

Save yourself

If the brain is the culprit in causing pain, can we use Jedi powers to brainwash it in some way to exert control or even think the pain away? Well, not entirely, but we can certainly hack the pain matrix in some ways. None of the tricks or hacks mentioned below are a guaranteed cure to prove the power of mind over body – not by any means. There are some pains that we just can't block in our current capacity so we will still be thwarted by vile gallstones and sickeningly painful tooth abscesses, unfortunately.

Get emotional Before we register pain, it goes through a factory line of signals until the brain processes it. These incoming signals from all over the body can be tweaked, influenced and even ramped up or down by the brain, creating bespoke pain just for you. In fact, your emotional state is involved in this process. For example, being sad or anxious about pain can heighten the experience. At the other end of the scale you have athletes who perform 'through the pain barrier' because they are so intensely focused and distracted from their pain that the nociceptive signals are briefly dampened.

This is a mind trick rooted in human physiology called descending pain modulation. It's the exact same reason why a placebo can provide analgesic effects. Just remember that while you can't think away or out-emote some pains, there are others that can be swayed by how much attention you give them and the situation you're in.

Look away One of the simplest mind tricks for dealing with pain is something I use on my patients all the time when taking blood. Just before I insert a cannula or even withdraw blood, I ask them to look away. The old adage 'out of sight, out of mind' is appropriate here because an external noxious stimulus can't be visualised. The brain is less sensitive to the pain as a result, which frees me up to get my work done without the poor patient passing out or throwing up. By shutting down a stimulus – visual in this case – it illustrates how influential the brain is in regulating pain. While looking away is an effective method for handling acute anticipated pain, sadly it doesn't work with chronic pain in which the tormentor lurks in the shadows and attacks without rhyme or reason.

KILLER INTELLIGENCE

I have ambivalent feelings about the human brain. It is undoubtedly responsible for us becoming the most dominant species on the planet and all the wonders of civilisation. Then again, people can be idiots. The best and worst of the brain is summed up by the word democracy; we built rockets and landed on the moon but we also sink into ice baths in winter and willingly eat kale.

Without doubt, the brain is one of the most complex things in the universe, and yet we are still only scratching the surface of what we think we know. For me, the fact that even after all these years there still remain mysteries of the human body is so exciting! If the brain were so simple that we could understand it all, chances are we would be too thick to comprehend it anyway.

Still, for all its prowess, I will always think of the brain as an absolute bastard. Occasionally, although thankfully now less common, it arrives in this world with murder in mind. The brain has killed millions of women through history on account of the size of the skull that is needed to house it. The brain's rapid expansion over millennia means our heads are now three times bigger than those of our closest cousins – the chimpanzee. This makes it altogether impractical for a woman's pelvic canal, which remains about the same size as one belonging to a female chimp. As a result, childbirth through history has proven to be an often fatal process.

Biologically and mathematically, modern humans have a far more perilous route into the world than other apes. They have to turn twice, as opposed to just once or not at all, when exiting their mother's womb. This increases the chances of arriving with the umbilical cord wrapped around their necks and, of course, increasing the chances of inadvertently killing their mothers through post-partum haemorrhage and various other obstetric complications. With childbirth, it has reached a point where we are now dependent on assistance to perform the most essential of biological functions.

Another issue is that our brains are not designed for the modern world. Our cultural progress has been incredibly rapid, which is ironic because our brains were biologically adapted to a very different world to the one we find ourselves in today. Things like motion sickness, cognitive biases, superstition, job stresses and obesity can be traced back to the fact that our brains still think we are hunter-gatherers on the plains of Africa.

It's fair to say that our culture and modern society has evolved at a faster pace than the brain. So, while it's still hard-wired for running away from wild beasts, it doesn't cope so well with the kind of stresses of modern life like mortgages and difficult bosses. Your line manager won't eat you for breakfast, but knowing they could fire you can be enough to leave you lying awake at night with worry. Yes, our brains might give rise to numerous mental health issues, which are often closely tied with modern living, but thankfully it still has a bright future. We just have to find ways to compensate for its shortcomings.

Brain 2.0 (release date delayed)

The brain claims to know the world around you. Since the dawn of humanity, it's convinced you that it's calling all the shots. In reality, it's just processing information that it's been fed by equally imperfect sensory organs. It's like a teenager, sitting in complete darkness playing on a computer racing simulation believing that they're really in the cockpit while keeping Lewis Hamilton in their wing mirrors.

Think about when you eat a mint and then breathe in. It feels cold, but why? Your brain is secretly combining information from thermal receptors activated by the chemical in the mint to construct a feeling of cold, but the temperature hasn't dropped by a single degree. Another is example is the feeling of being wet; this is an illusion because humans don't have specific wetness receptors. When you feel wet, moist, sweaty, humid . . . that's a form of perceptual illusion. Your brain just patches together different senses and associates that feeling with wetness. It combines your ability to detect cold temperature with tactile sensations like pressure and texture and adds this information to your existing knowledge of things that you have learned are wet: a damp towel or some dribble on the toilet seat as it touches your butt cheeks. Your brain literally fools you into feeling this 'wetness' but this simulation is imperfect; that's why it's sometimes hard to tell if your towel is actually wet or just really cold.

The reality you sense around you is heavily redacted and filtered by your brain so you only experience what's important. What's more, your brain doesn't stop there. It constantly makes complex calculations to estimate and predict what will happen next, using stored data and past experiences to guide your actions. It doesn't simply react to the world, it is calling upon predictive modelling and preparing your actions in anticipation of the event, and before receiving sensory data. So, when a ball is thrown at your face, your brain has already taken steps ahead of your conscious thought to move out of the way. This happens so imperceptibly fast that you don't notice such efficient forward-planning.

Having recognised the flaws of our brain, and the ways it compensates for itself as much as own ability to adapt to its shortcomings, we can perhaps hope for improvements as new operating systems drop. Right now, advances in artificial intelligence are giving rise to algorithmic learning systems that can do our thinking for us. First they come for our chess trophies. Soon, they'll be sitting in our driving seats and taking over our surgical operations and . . . hey, wait!

The future might seem uncertain, but we can only hope that man and machine will come together to enhance our brains for the greater good. We could even see the functions of our wrinkled, grey blancmanges uploaded on to cloud-based networks. In time, our computer-enhanced brains may even shed light on the full workings of the old model, and I for one will activate my synthesised voice box and declare: 'They don't make them like that anymore.'

[Half Page Illustration To Come]

Health Hack

Here's a quick and easy way to slow down neurodegeneration, the term used to describe how your brain and central nervous system lose their performance edge with age.

* Regular exercise improves blood flow to the brain, keeping you sharp into later life.

* Sleep clears away toxic proteins that accumulate in the brain through your busy day.

* Social interaction is known to keep the brain engaged, which means making friends is a smart move.

* It's never too late to challenge yourself! Try learning a new language or take up a musical instrument to reduce the risk of developing dementia.

* Do something that fills you with wonder and awe. Whether it's a simple walk surrounded by nature to gazing at the stars and contemplating the meaning of your existence, studies show that blowing your mind can help to keep the brain firing on all cylinders long into old age.

3. The Bloody Chamber

A HOT TAKE ON
THE HEART

THE HEART IS DEEPLY INTERTWINED with the initiation of life. Six
weeks after conception, it is the first organ that develops in the womb,
when a group of cells come together and say, 'hey let's start dancing
together' and beat in sync.

Much like all living creatures, your muscular heart serves to pump oxygen
and nutrient parcels around the body via arteries. In driving the flow of
blood through the veins, it's also key in removing waste products like
carbon dioxide.

The heart is unflagging and selfless, never taking a break, so you can
sleep at night knowing that someone or something is keeping guard and
ensuring you live to see the next day. Most of you will have the luxury of
experiencing roughly 3 billion heartbeats in a lifetime. It works tirelessly to
keep you alive with the kind of reliability that mechanical engineers could
never match. If it did stop momentarily, the entire body would lose its
oxygen supply. That's a big responsibility.

When you're resting, your heart pumps around 5 litres of blood around
the body every minute. In a fit and healthy individual, it can also amplify
this volume by a factor of eight or nine. Yet despite working so hard,
the heart isn't a selfish organ. It consumes only 5 per cent of your entire

blood flow. Essentially, your heart is the thoroughbred horse of the body, destined to perform one purpose as efficiently and dependably as possible. Your heart cells cannot regenerate and respawn. This means that when you eventually die you take with you 50 per cent of the cardiac cells you were born with. Your heart is so strong-willed that if you were to remove it from your body it would continue to beat on its own; one could say this is a testament to its relentless worth ethic. Not only is it an incredible pump and electrical circuit rolled into one, but the heart also plays a central role in all of human culture from literature, art and music to love. It's the organ that means everything to everyone.

A lifetime allowance

One of the most popular urban myths about the heart is that humans have a set number of beats before it expires. This isn't a totally bizarre concept. The heart of the blue whale beats just 8 times per minute, while in that same time the little Etruscan shrew hammers in at over 800, and yet all mammals great and small experience the same average number of heartbeats in a lifetime, which amounts to about half a billion. This is known as *the rate of living* hypothesis, and yet it doesn't apply to humans. Why not? Because advances in hygiene, medicine and science have allowed us to break beyond these hypothetical constraints and extend the number of heartbeats we enjoy compared to other mammals.

So, that's all the flattery I have to offer about the heart. Now it's time to dig into the downsides.

FAILINGS OF THE HUMAN HEART

The excesses of modern society, bad luck, bad habits and sometimes an unfortunate genetic inheritance can all act to break your heart. Plaque, which is basically biological debris, can accumulate in your arteries; this is akin to your body fly-tipping rubbish in forbidden areas as an act of defiance against high levels of cholesterol. We're talking about the bad stuff that accumulates (atherosclerotic plaque) as a result of smoking, not exercising enough and dietary factors, although it's occasionally due to genetics. All these factors contribute to heart disease, which is the biggest and often most insidious killer of humans.

In the UK, heart disease contributes to more than a quarter of all adult deaths. This amounts to a kill count of about one every 3 minutes. So why is this vital pump so prone to being bullied, and how does it fail us?

Feel the pump

The heart is a muscle-bound and oxygen-hungry organ. You'd think it would be guaranteed a reliable and generous blood supply, and yet in reality it's somewhat pathetic. Rather than a gleaming manifold to manage flow, the heart is fitted with two little arteries, about 3mm in diameter. If one becomes blocked, which is a very common thing to happen to your body, it's called a heart attack. This slip-up seems unique to the human heart; other animals show it doesn't have to be this way. Dogs for example, have some collateral supplies. This means if they experience a heart attack it's mitigated by a tree-like network of smaller blood vessels which branch out from the main coronary arteries. Think of it as a handy diversion to your destination if the main road is closed.

Human hearts have very limited coronary collateral supplies, which isn't ideal if the main blood pipes are injured or blocked in any way. Stimulating the growth of collateral blood vessels could help combat insufficient blood flow and reduce the risk of heart attacks, but this is very much at a research stage in medical science. While we wait for the invention of an immortal heart, or a virtual world we actually want to inhabit, there is one free and easy way to mitigate the flaws in your heart's engineering, and that's exercise.

We can rebuild it

Your blood vessels have an internal lining of cells called endothelial cells and physical activity creates a little bit of magic. The endothelial cells release nitric oxide, the same stuff that appears in toxic fumes from the tailpipes of cars that have failed their MOT. In small amounts, however, this environmental pollutant is actually a godsend for your circulatory system. It has two key roles. The first is to keep the lining of your arteries slippery and smooth; this enables your white blood cells and platelets to enjoy a bump-free ride so they don't stick and cause pipe-blocking blood clots. Secondly, nitric oxide relaxes the smooth muscles present in the middle layer of your arteries and keeps them nice and wide, which improves blood flow. In fact, it is exactly this mechanism of boosting the endothelial cells' nitric oxide production that led doctors to create Viagra, which works by bringing more blood to the penis, thus producing an erection.

The little blue pill

Viagra was never intended as a trouser-raising drug. It was originally developed in 1989 as the drug UK-92480 by Pfizer scientists who were looking into a treatment for angina, a heart-related chest pain. The hypothesis was that this drug would block the enzyme PDE5, thus causing vessels to widen to increase blood flow and lower blood pressure. However, this medication – known as sildenafil citrate – had a curious side effect. One vigilant nurse noted that volunteers of this drug trial were lying on their stomachs due to embarrassing and unexpected erections. Scientists quickly realised the potential of this and turned a side effect into a multibillion-dollar enterprise to tackle erectile dysfunction.

As an aside, poor heart health and reduced blood flow can be a factor when it comes to erectile dysfunction. The good news is that exercise is considered to be an effective antidote – with broader benefits beyond the bedroom – that allows heart vessels to grow tiny new blood vessels. This is a unique process known as angiogenesis, which can improve blood supply and help to stave off heart disease. Think of it as a form of pseudo-auto bypass surgery giving you some of the benefits of bypass surgery minus the scars. You can develop angiogenesis from aerobic exercise such as hiking, running, cycling and swimming, or even just walking and adding regularity to your workouts.

Sprint finish

Legend has it that when the Athenians found out the Persians had arrived in the town of Marathon during their invasion of Greece in 490 BC, a messenger by the name Pheidippides ran to Sparta bearing a request for assistance. Perhaps the first and original 'marathon' runner, he covered 260 kilometres in under two days and promptly collapsed and died immediately afterwards. History doesn't record whether Pheidippides died of a heart attack but scientists are now investigating what effect extreme exercise has on the heart.

Thankfully most of us do not need to worry about being too fit; rather the opposite. However, extreme endurance athletes like ultra-marathon runners can develop various heart rhythm abnormalities and heart damage. The theory is that extreme endurance activities burdens the cardiovascular system, resulting in the heart being structurally 'remodelled': the walls of the heart become thicker and scar tissue builds up. These physical changes may lead to irregular heartbeats like atrial fibrillation. As with anything, the poison is in the dose. Too much of a good thing might end up being bad for you.

It's not just 'extreme' exercise that can compromise the heart but also the type of exercise undertaken by young, elite-level athletes. Increasingly over the past few decades a number of footballers have died suddenly while playing the game they love, all seemingly fit and healthy. This isn't down to bad luck or a mysterious coincidence that could give rise to a web of conspiracy theories. It's associated with a deadly condition known as hypertrophic obstructive cardiomyopathy (HOCM). This causes the heart of young athletes to behave like that of an eighty-year-old. The intensely exercised hearts of these young sporting professionals are moulded according to the stress of their training. Initially, this structural heart renovation is useful; it creates a pump that is more efficient to meet the increased demands the body requires. If you suffer from HOCM, however, it's not so good. The condition is down to a genetic abnormality that causes the muscular wall of the heart to grow far thicker than required. Excessive training results in a wall so thick it can impede the proper flow of blood, which is where things can get disastrous. You might think this is rare, but HOCM is surprisingly common. It affects approximately 1 in 500 people, though most aren't elite sporting stars and will live their life symptom free.

For an athlete, the first sign of trouble may turn out to be the last sign. A sudden cardiac arrest can be fatal. If the heart stops, technically the person is deceased. The only real chance they have at a second life depends on whether anyone is present capable of performing cardiopulmonary resuscitation, or CPR.

The face of CPR and Michael Jackson

Let me take you back to late nineteenth-century Paris and the story of L'Inconnue de la Seine (the unknown woman of the Seine). While she will never know of her posthumous fame, the young lady in question transformed the face of medical emergency training that would lead to millions of lives being saved.

In the late 1880s, the body of an adolescent girl was found in the river Seine. The body was sent to the morgue and the tale could have simply ended here. With no means by which to identify her, the corpse was left on display in the mortuary in the hope it might be recognised by family members. In doing so, the duty pathologist became deeply enchanted by her enigmatic half-smile and eerily serene appearance. He went so far as to commission a plaster cast 'death mask' of her visage to immortalise this beautiful expression. Very soon the mask captured the imagination of more than just the pathologist. In fact, it became widely replicated and sold as a decorative piece for people's homes. Yes, death masks were statements of interior decoration back then, and the dead Parisian girl quickly became known as L'Inconnue de la Seine.

Jump forward to the 1960s, where Austrian doctor Peter Safar had already developed a rudimentary form of mouth-to-mouth CPR. Understandably, medical students found this first aid difficult to practise on each other so Safar reached out to a Belgian toymaker called Asmund Laerdal to produce a teaching mannequin. In his search for a lifelike face, Laerdal recalled a death mask he had seen in his grandparents' house when he was younger, which is how L'Inconnue de la Seine became the face of the training mannequin. The dummy was called 'Resusci Anne' or 'CPR Annie' and became the tool through which millions of people, perhaps even you, learned CPR. As a result, Annie holds the honourable title of being the most kissed girl in the world. Michael Jackson even referenced her in the lyrics of his song 'Smooth Criminal' by asking, 'Annie, are you OK?', a phrase that CPR students have long been taught to use when initially assessing their unresponsive plastic patient.

Hollywood gets it wrong

My first ever shift as a doctor also ended up being the first time I witnessed death in front of my eyes. It was 11am and the automated message on my emergency bleep sounded: 'cardiac arrest, ward E1, cardiac arrest, ward E1'. As I ran with my senior to the room of a patient who was previously reported to have trouble breathing, I was greeted with an overwhelming smell of vomit, the inescapable feeling of foreboding and a cluster of doctors, healthcare assistants and nurses crowded around the patient. The elderly lady had a glass-eyed stare while her body jolted under repeated chest compressions. It was enough to produce a knot in my throat.

When a patient has suffered a cardiopulmonary arrest, and their heart is no longer beating, they are technically dead. It's the human version of a power outage. This is different from a heart attack, which is usually due to a plumbing problem, in which one of the coronary arteries is blocked, rather than an electrical malfunction. Both are emergency situations and indeed a heart attack is a common cause for a cardiac arrest. When electrical activity ceases in the heart, and blood is no longer spontaneously moving, chest compressions are essentially a means of keeping the heart pumping manually. It's an attempt to maintain blood flow to vital organs along with the hope that the heart will return to spontaneous heart activity or come back with the assistance of a defibrillator.

I relieved one of the nurses who was performing CPR and began compressing the patient's chest. She was ninety years old and frail. I could hear her ribs breaking under the weight of my CPR. I felt sick.

I'd only ever performed CPR on dummies or seen it on TV. In real life, all the training and viewing can suddenly seem quite meaningless. Poor form and technique aside, Hollywood has misinformed the public about the success rates and outcomes after CPR. Film and TV portrays it as a highly successful heroic manoeuvre. Sadly, this is not the case; the survival rate of cardiac arrest patients to discharge is somewhere around 20 per cent. For out of hospital cardiac arrests, that number drops precipitously to single digits.

In some cases, us medics have another tool up our sleeve if CPR alone isn't working. It's also a Hollywood favourite, in which the heroic doctor applies two defibrillator pads to the patient's chest and shocks them back to life. In reality, defibrillators don't restart a non-beating heart. They actually turn it off in the hope that it'll reboot on its own and escape the abnormal rhythm. Shocking a patient with a flat line on a heart monitor accomplishes nothing, unless you plan to have your meat well done. When someone enters a state of cardiac arrest, they might need to be shocked depending on the rhythm and if it is a 'shockable' rhythm or not. A flat line falls into the unshockable side. The most common heart rhythm in a cardiac arrest is known as ventricular fibrillation – a fluttering of the heart – and this is appropriate to shock.

With my elderly patient showing some faint sign of heart activity on the monitor, we continued several rounds of CPR before moving on to more desperate measures. Unfortunately, she did not pull through despite two shots of adrenaline and several defibrillator shocks. As her time of death was announced, I had to remind myself that such efforts are always worthwhile, even if there is no guaranteed outcome. Despite seeing several more cardiac arrests after that one, I couldn't shake the feeling of helplessness. It stayed with me for years, in fact, and brought back vivid memories as I watched the Euro 2020 match on TV between

Denmark and Finland, when the Danish player, Christian Eriksen, collapsed to the ground minutes before the end of the first half with what was later revealed as a cardiac arrest. Fortunately, due to quick action from players and staff, he received early CPR and resuscitative efforts. Such was his recovery that Eriksen still continues to play at the highest level of football. Thanks to the wonders of medicine and technology, he has a mini pacemaker device implanted around his heart that picks up abnormal heart rhythms and reverses them before they become lethal.

The appendage you don't know about

If I were to invite you to guess the name of an appendage that exists inside the body, a little redundant pocket of tissue that is about the size of your little finger but which invariably causes people to get sick and maybe even die, I bet most of you would say the appendix. Given that we now know that this little guy plays a key role in populating the gut flora, however, in this case you would be wrong

I'm talking about a truly villainous appendage that causes way more harm – and in some cases even death – than the appendix could ever hope to achieve. It goes by the name of the left atrial appendage, which comes off the heart and is responsible for about a quarter of all strokes.

On paper, blood clotting seems like a good idea, and a better option than uncontrollable bleeding. In reality, when clotting takes place inside the body and in the wrong place, it can cause all manner of problems. I'm sure you've heard about people getting clots in their legs or in their lungs; in fact, most heart attacks are typically blood clots in the heart. These often come from the left atrial appendage and are caused by an irregular heart rhythm, also called atrial fibrillation, and it's pretty common as we get older. With an irregular rhythm, the blood starts to pool in that little appendage. Eventually, it solidifies into a blood clot and before you know it it's gone up to the brain and you've had a stroke. This dastardly appendage, infamous for harbouring murderous fugitive blood clots and giving them safe passage to the rest of your circulation, is surely a menace to your body. It serves no good purpose other than to be a medical curiosity with potentially deadly consequences.

A heart full of holes

Brace yourselves for a scary fact: there's a 25 per cent chance that you're living with a hole in the heart. In the vast majority of cases this doesn't cause problems. It's considered to be a normal variant and serves as an accidental biological doorway between your left and right atrium. Usually, the left side and the right side of the heart shouldn't have any gaps between them (once you're born) and in most cases this hole is absolutely tiny. It's basically a remnant of the insanely complicated way that the heart forms when you're developing in the womb.

While most holes are harmless, other faults can develop with a range of consequences from manageable to catastrophic. One of the ways of managing this fault involves an extra tube we all have called the left internal mammary artery. This runs from the subclavian artery in your neck/upper shoulder junction and connects to your chest wall. If you disconnect one end it doesn't really cause any problems, so some clever person had the idea to stick that loose end on to the heart as a substitute when other pipes are at risk of packing in, and called it a coronary artery bypass operation. So, next time you're tucking into your fried chips just be thankful that your body is fitted with a backup kit should your heart require it.

Broken heart club

So far we've spoken about all the tangible ways in which your heart can ruin your life but what about a broken heart? When you see this phrase you most likely imagine a cartoon heart comically cracking like a piece of fine china. What if I told you that your heart can actually 'break', even causing you to die? The fact is that broken heart syndrome is more literal than figurative.

During periods of emotional upheaval, such as the breakdown of a long-term relationship or a bereavement, your body can experience elevated levels of stress hormones. In turn, this can lead to a stress-induced cardiomyopathy or takotsubo cardiomyopathy, a weakening of the heart muscle. The condition is named after the Japanese term 'tako-tsubo' which is a vase-like octopus trap – the shape the heart adopts during this condition.

Takotsubo cardiomyopathy can start suddenly and without warning, even in healthy individuals. Signs include chest pain, shortness of breath, abnormal ECG readings – basically typical things you would find in a heart attack except for blocked coronary arteries. Oddly enough, the strong emotions don't have to be purely negative. Around 1 per cent of broken heart syndrome cases are initiated by positive events like the birth of a baby, which can lead to intense feelings at the other side of the scale. Ultimately, death from a broken heart is rare but yes, you can have your heart broken and it can be fatal.

THE HAPPY HEART

Considering all the ways it can kill us – both torturously slowly and with ninja-like speed and skill – how do we fight back against the heart and perhaps even turn it into an ally so that we can live longer, fulfilling lives? We know that a sensible diet and moderate, regular exercise are major factors, but what about the smart hacks that can help our hearts?

Be fat informed

It might seem peculiar that what we eat can have such a profound effect on the heart, given that is processed predominantly by our far-removed gastrointestinal system, but diet is increasingly recognised as a key factor in its health.

We know that a high intake of fibre isn't just protective for the gut, but it can also help to lower blood pressure and cholesterol levels. Paradoxically, fat can play an important role in keeping your ticker in good shape. Ensuring an adequate intake of fatty acids like omega-3 can reduce the levels of triglycerides, a type of fat found in the blood, thus reducing your blood pressure and blood clot risk. Omega-3 found in fatty fish, for example, plays an important role in the creation of hormones that maintain good artery health. Walnuts, almonds and various other nuts are also beneficial, along with fruit that is high in pectin (a plant-based source of omega-3).

Save yourself

In order to keep the heart from staging an unwelcome strike, we should limit our consumption of both saturated fatty acids and in particular trans fats, found in high amounts in processed meats and foods. Then we come to salt, which is a key compound involved in regulating our blood pressure and indirectly heart health. It is difficult to live a life devoid of salt and neither would this be recommended. In the modern world, however, the foods we consume – in particular the ultra-processed variety – have inordinate amounts of added salt. On current evidence we should look to limit our salt intake to under 5g a day. If you are a ravenous carnivore, I wouldn't for one moment dream of trying to convert you to veganism or vegetarianism – because I don't fall into either group. Nevertheless, a reduction in red meat intake can only help to lower cholesterol and promote good heart health.

Stress

This is a sneaky one. Some stress is actually good for us; it literally gets our juices flowing, increases our heart rate and allows for more efficient circulating of blood. It's also a natural consequence and prelude to exercise and intense activity. However, chronic, unyielding stress can be harmful. Persistent stresses, such as at work or in a relationship, can flood your biological systems with stress hormones like cortisol. This is enough to dysregulate your blood sugar, cause systemic low-grade inflammation and persistently raise your blood pressure – all of which are clearly not amenable to good heart health.

Blood pressure

Your blood pressure is a marker of how hard your heart is working. Uncontrolled high blood pressure, known as hypertension, is akin to turning a blind eye to slave labour. In this case, you've unwittingly overworked your heart, who will return the favour in kind when you least suspect.

Prolonged periods of hypertension can put mechanical stress on the walls of the arteries, causing them to change shape, harden and even narrow. In turn this becomes the perfect breeding ground for heart attacks and strokes. This increased stress can trigger plaque formation – biological speedbumps in your arteries – and cause the heart muscle to both weaken and also thicken over time.

When you see blood pressure readings, you often see a fraction, e.g. 120/80. The top number is the systolic pressure, which represents the contraction of the heart, and the lower number is the diastolic pressure when your heart is at rest and filling. It is perfectly normal for blood pressure to rise slightly with increasing age – and age-related degeneration of the circulatory system – but keeping those numbers in check is crucial as hypertension is a leading cause for heart attacks as well as stroke.

Your blood pressure fluctuates throughout the day. It can be influenced by poor sleep, stress, caffeine, alcohol and emotions. Ideally you want to measure it on at least two occasions or more to get an accurate average. The importance of controlling high blood pressure is so critical that studies have illustrated that for every decrease of ten of your systolic blood pressure, your stroke risk goes down by 27 per cent and your risk of heart disease by 17 per cent.

Save yourself

While a working knowledge of the heart and its fragilities can cause enough anxiety to induce a cardiac arrest, how do you actually lower blood pressure? Much is achieved with lifestyle changes to promote a healthy heart, such as moderating your alcohol intake, limiting salt to under 5g a day and getting some exercise under your belt.

In addition, one of the largest heart studies, the Framingham Heart Study, found that excess body weight was the culprit for roughly a quarter of hypertension cases in men and up to a third of cases in women. It makes sense: the more load you carry on your frame, the harder your heart has to work to get blood to your entire body. So occasionally, in a select group of people, weight reduction as an adjunct to other factors can be a key step towards reining in your blood pressure.

Cholesterol

Cholesterol is a type of fat, or lipid, found in the blood and is one of many factors that has an integral role in shaping the health of your circulatory and cardiovascular system. It's important to understand but can also be quite a complex, in that not all cholesterol can be considered bad.

In short, high-density lipoprotein cholesterol (HDL) is considered protective, and is found in antioxidant foods like nuts and berries, while low-density lipoprotein cholesterol (LDL) is the 'bad' guy, found in fatty cuts of meat or full-fat dairy products. Things aren't quite that simple, but in effect higher HDL and lower LDL levels are commensurate with better cardiovascular health.

We also have triglycerides. These are a type of calorie-converted fat circulating in the bloodstream, and we call on it for energy. Consuming a sugar-rich diet, or simply glugging a sports drink, can increase levels of triglycerides, which is effectively fuel for the body. So, in moderation, and in combination with physical activity, we're talking about a fat that can serve an important purpose.

Excess weight – and particularly fat – plays a hidden role in poor heart health. Basically, as more fat accumulates in your body, a chain of hormonal changes occur that culminate in the release of pesky chemicals called adipokines, which can influence blood sugar levels, blood pressure and the concentration of fat globules in the blood. These go hand in glove with inflammatory changes in blood vessels, which act to hasten the development of stiffer arteries, arterial damage, high blood pressure and chronic heart disease.

In many cases, high cholesterol can be managed with diet, exercise and lifestyle changes but it may not always be enough as there is a significant genetic component in this too.

Blood sugar

Your blood sugar level is another key aspect worth monitoring and is can be a risk factor for heart disease when left unchecked. Exercise and a nutritious diet will go a long way to regulating levels. However, there are some surprising elements that can subtly contribute to chronically elevated blood glucose levels. The good news is they are avoidable.

Getting plenty of good shuteye is our first port of call. Poor sleep can contribute to insulin resistance and elevate your blood glucose. Then we have alcohol, which can leave levels like a storm drain after a downpour. Another insidious culprit is chronic stress. This triggers the hormone cortisol, which can increase blood sugar levels.

[Half Page Illustration To Come]

Health Hack

Heartburn is another name for acid reflux. It has nothing to do with your ticker – even though it can feel like it's on fire – but a term used to describe that feeling when stomach juices travel upwards towards the throat. It's uncomfortable and unpleasant, but the good news is that you can minimise the chances of it happening by cutting down or even avoiding certain foods.

* Onions are a rich source of fermentable fibre, which can result in increased burping. This can stir up stomach acids and cause it to head against the traffic.

* Limit high fat foods because they stimulate the release of the hormone cholecystokinin. This can cause the lower oesophageal sphincter to relax, increasing the risk of acid reflux.

* Be wary of spicy food. This is because it often contains capsaicin, a chemical that slows the rate of digestion so that food sits in the stomach for longer and increases the risk of heartburn.

4. Airway to Heaven

THE LETHALITY OF LUNGS

THE GREATEST FLAW OF THE LUNGS is arguably there through no fault of its own. Compared to other body parts, it is terribly starved of attention. Until recently, we just took the lungs for granted, which means it is markedly underfunded when it comes to disease research compared with other health conditions. Then the Covid-19 virus stopped the world from turning for a time, which prompted us to mask up to protect this pair of precious organs as if our lives depended on it.

For all its beauty (as well as crimes), the heart would be nothing without its sidekick – and occasional deadly assassin. The lungs are the only twin organs in the body that refuse to function in utero, which is probably for the best. They also mark the beginning of independent life with a scream and gasp of air as the two caskets, now drained of fluid, inflate for the very first time.

With 20,000 or so breaths taken every day to allow oxygen to permeate through and nourish the cells in your body, you are so reliant on breathing that if it stopped you would die within minutes. It's just something that happens in the background, under the radar of your conscious awareness most of the time, but mostly reliable and adaptable to your requirements.

About 300 million years ago, our water-dwelling ancestors dragged themselves on to the land and made a commitment to surface breathing. Even since, we've been paying the price. The lungs are basically two big balloons, filled with mucus and millions of tiny air sacs. To be fair, most of the time they work in a synchronised fashion, allowing you to savour the breath of life. It's a perpetual engine much like the heart . . . except for the times when it malfunctions. You only have to have an anxiety attack, find yourself choked off by a headlock or a crumb of food in your windpipe, and then the lungs lose their proverbial shit.

The lungs are the understated workhorse of the body. As well as perfecting the art of extracting air from the outside world, they also dump the waste products created by your tissues, like carbon dioxide, and trade this in like a 24-hour recycling centre.

AND BREATHE

There is something strange, almost mystical, about the lungs. The ayurvedic practitioners of ancient India, and proponents of traditional Eastern medicine, believed that the air you breathed carried life energy and spirit. They called it prana and qi respectively. For this same reason, gurus and mystics in the foothills of the Himalayas entrenched themselves in deep meditation and intense breathing practices in a bid to transcend their corporeal form and blur the thin interface between the spiritual and physical world.

There's an undeniable link between how you breathe and your state of mind. In a chicken/egg-type situation, it is sometimes difficult to determine what comes first. Unlike the heart, whose rhythm is governed by specialised pacemaker cells, your lungs and the surrounding breathing muscles take their orders directly from the brain. Despite the significance of this, it took us until the 1980s to figure out the exact origin of the lungs' controlling signals. While the ancient Greek physician, Galen, noted that gladiators with broken necks at specific levels of the cervical region of the spinal cord had issues breathing, it wasn't until centuries later than Jack Feldman and colleagues identified a few thousand neurons in the human brainstem, called the pre-Bötzinger complex, as being responsible for directing the orchestra of breathing.

Without doubt, breathing is something we take for granted. We're talking about an invisible process, after all, and not many of us have the privilege of an inside view to appreciate just what an incredible structure the lungs have shaped up to be. The thing that struck me most about them, when I first cracked open a cadaver's chest in the anatomy lab, was not their ethereal power but how perfectly moulded they were to the shape of the chest cavity. They could be factory-fitted, similar to those integral parts in modern appliances like washing machines and televisions that can't be replaced when they break.

One of the first things you get taught in medical school, on pressing the chilled stethoscope head to the naked chest and back of a patient, is the various breath sounds heard in disease states compared to the normal variants. Despite having all manner of tools and fancy scans, the tried-and-tested stethoscope stands the test of time to detect the pathology. On one particular night shift (my third of four in a row), I reviewed a patient who had driven his car into a tree; the tree won. He had suspected rib fractures and I proceeded to urgently examine his chest to see if he had any evidence of a collapsed lung. This is known as a pneumothorax. Fractured ribs can often pierce the membrane surrounding the lungs. This allows air to leak into the space between the lung and chest wall, causing the patient to become increasingly agitated and short of breath.

Listening through my stethoscope, I detected a worrying absence of breath sounds in his left lung. When I percussed (tapped) on this left lung it was like a drum (hyperresonant, since you ask). This was indicative of a potentially fatal lung collapse with the air compressing the lung, known as a tension pneumothorax. I'd actually never seen one in person, but from my medical textbook knowledge I knew what I had to do. I stabbed a cannula into his upper chest and was greeted with a relieving hiss of air escaping from the chest cavity. At once, the patient's laboured breathing began to settle. A chest X-ray revealed the other side had a hemothorax, a bleed into the lung space also due to fractured ribs.

As quickly as I could, I gathered an assortment of equipment: a chest drain (a plastic tube to drain blood), a scalpel, some local anaesthetic, plenty of gauze and some stitches. Over the next 10 minutes, with some grunting and groaning from both of us, I positioned chest drains into the patient's left and right lungs. In response, I was greeted with a fountain of blood which siphoned off into the right-hand drain. After 500ml had drained out, the patient appeared more comfortable, less short of breath and mildly hungry. You would too after losing half a litre of blood.

Oxygen mechanics

The engineering behind lung function is both highly impressive and insultingly basic. With each inhalation, the diaphragm muscle contracts and moves downwards. At the same time, the intercostal muscles between the ribs (you'll recognise these if you're a fan of barbecue) move your ribcage upwards and outwards. This coordination helps to draw air in. Exhalation is more of a passive process that occurs when these muscles relax and the lungs gently deflate with a sigh.

There is one quite obvious problem with this set-up. Every time you take a breath in, with the hope of getting some nice fresh air into your lungs, it mixes with the stale air remaining in your respiratory system. This means by the time it gets to the air sacs for gas exchange it's partly stale. Think about when you swig the last mouthful of water from a bottle . . . you know it's mainly saliva and backwash, right? In your lungs, a constant level of stale air contaminates each new inhale, only this 'respiratory backwash' is called dead space.

This is one of the reasons why you have a large respiratory network to get through rapid oxygen and carbon dioxide exchange when demands are high. It's also why you can 'run out' of breath under heavy exertion. Just when you need it most, your lungs fail you and limit your abilities. Thankfully, it doesn't mean you get gobbled up by the neighbourhood sabretooth tiger anymore. You just miss that bus and end up late for work.

In suggesting the lungs work like a pair of balloons, I should admit that I am doing them a slight disservice. The mechanics of breathing are slightly more nuanced than a mindless pump which pulls in and pushes out gases. The lungs are bursting with immune cells. They also play a role in maintaining the pH levels of your blood in tandem with the kidneys. With each inhalation, the air descends through labyrinthine internal catacombs in each lung that would cover upwards of a thousand miles if re-formed into a line. Thankfully, given the distance, this is mostly automated by the brainstem.

The millions of microscopic air sacs inside the lungs are collectively called alveoli. These form the crux of the respiratory system where gas exchange occurs. Each alveolus, the width of a human hair, is surrounded by a mesh of micro-capillaries that carry oxygen to the rest of the bloodstream and return carbon dioxide to be vented with each exhalation. There's a lot riding on this exchange process. In fact, your life depends on it. While the immediacy of the effect it carries is remarkable, allowing oxygen to be diffused into the bloodstream at mind boggling speeds, it must also draw out noxious gases that could otherwise enter the brain with equal efficiency and lead to your demise.

You might think your reason for breathing is simply down to a hunger for oxygen but in fact this is only a kernel of the truth. The primary drive for breathing is your body's abhorrence of too much carbon dioxide, which can turn your blood acidic when it accumulates.

Butthole breathing

In considering the importance of gas exchange in the lungs, it's not unreasonable to ask why your mouth and nose have to do all the work. After all, you're fitted with another pink and fleshy orifice that with some modification could serve as a backup oxygen generator. At present, nature dictates that your anus has just one job. We can all agree it would be remarkable if your butthole could also breathe for you, and not just because you'd be set up for life with the ultimate party trick. It might sound like a dream, but the fact is that scientists in Japan have recently found out that pigs and rodents absorb oxygen through their anuses, and can even survive without breathing through the lungs. It's an incredible superpower, but perhaps one that might test the marketing department.

Invaders must die

This main entry portal into your precious air real estate also happens to be one of your biggest weak points. You have the misfortune of sharing a breathing hole, your trachea, with a feeding inlet. As a result, every time you eat or drink something you're unwittingly playing Choke Roulette. To add to this further, the insides of the lungs are so sensitive that any food or liquid substances that enter the lungs via the trachea can trigger an uncomfortable, and sometimes even serious, chemical response. In a hospital setting, I often see this when a patient inhales their vomit or secretions after surgery, or after an unexpectedly violent episode of retching. This can result in a chemical inflammation of the lung known as aspiration pneumonia.

Even if you successfully avoid dropping food down your windpipe, or trachea, it's still an open gateway for insidious pathogens, irritant pollutants and irksome allergens to enter and cause havoc for your breathing.

When your lungs aren't becoming irate on detecting non-air substances touching their insides, they occasionally go into military mode, for example when battling a viral or bacterial assault. Such an invasion can leave your lungs filled to the brim with mucus, resulting in heavy, laboured breathing. Worse still, if you're an asthmatic then your lungs might decide to choke themselves and leave you breathless when provoked by even the most innocuous of things – cold air, dust or even cigarette smoke.

The lungs may seem hardy, but in reality they are incredibly fragile. The accumulation of microscopic scars from smoking, inflammation or infection can damage the collagen and elastic fibres in the alveoli. This deprives them of elasticity and recoil, resulting in chronic lung disease.

In a bid to reduce your risk of basically dying with every breath you take, the lungs also serve as air purifiers. They work by trapping particulate matter in a mucus lining and then transporting it upwards for rejection. This is carried out by millions of tiny hair like projections called cilia. Coating the airways, they beat furiously to redirect invading particles back through the oesophagus. If they're not swallowed into the stomach along the way, they might arrive with coughing, sneezing or retching into your mouth. Tasty.

Assisted breathing

The Covid pandemic highlighted the need to expand our options when it comes to breathing. Mechanical ventilation, in which air is artificially pushed into the lungs through the windpipe, is our current default when the lungs need help. Then we have extracorporeal membrane oxygenation (ECMO), in which blood is pumped out of the body and reoxygenated in artificial lungs.

The basic concept of an artificial breathing mechanism has been in existence for decades. In the nineteenth century, patients were required to sit upright in airtight chambers with their heads poking out. The internal air pressure of the chamber would be increased or decreased by a pair of bellows that had to be manually worked from the outside. This ultimately caused a compression or expansion of the patient's chest cavity to mimic natural breathing. It was these early forms of 'negative pressure ventilators' that led to the invention of the dreaded – but ultimately lifesaving – iron lung.

In the early twentieth century, polio was one of the most feared diseases. The virus could lead to respiratory paralysis, making breathing impossible. In the 1940s and 1950s, it was a leading cause of childhood and adolescent death, which made a spell inside the iron lung a little more tolerable for young patients.

These behemoths were giant ventilators that sometimes measured up to 7 feet long. A child afflicted with polio, and therefore barely able to breathe unassisted, would be entombed up to the neck within the lung. A pair of bellows at the foot of the device would mirror the function of the human diaphragm. This forced air in and out of the patient's lungs via negative and positive pressure respectively.

The iron lung could be a deeply unpleasant experience for the patient encased inside, and yet the device assisted breathing for long enough to defeat the virus and breathe independently within a few weeks. Disturbingly, there are a few notable cases of patients who never recovered the ability to breathe on their own, and were forced to spend their entire lives trapped inside this metal cage. In the latter half of the twentieth century, the advent of an effective vaccination programme practically eradicated the virus from the developed world, which also spelled an end to this dreaded but necessary form of ventilation.

Save yourself

As you're old enough to read, you might think it's too late to learn how to breathe properly. For the most part, it's an involuntary process, the rate of which is governed by the brainstem. Even so, we have some conscious control over it and you can learn to breathe better with some basic tips and tricks.

An understated facet of good breathing is your posture. Correct posture means your diaphragm isn't constricted. This means ensuring you back is upright, while your shoulders aren't hunched forward but depressed and rolled back slightly. Have your chin slightly tilted up, with your jaw, neck and shoulders loosely relaxed.

While you do that, just take a moment to consider your mouth and shut it if needs be. I don't mean that in an offensive way. The issue is that most of us are chronic mouth breathers and this can dry out the mouth, leading to halitosis. It can also irritate your lungs as well as be a causative factor in sleep apnoea too. Using your nose rather than mouth to breathe in takes advantage of the natural filters built into your body.

It helps to filter, humidify and clean the air before it enters your sensitive internal environment. Nasal breathing allows for deeper, richer breaths. The stresses of modern life can often disengage you from effective diaphragmatic breathing. Instead, it pushes us towards less refreshing, shallower, chest breathing. You can try for yourself now: lie on your back on a bed with your knees slightly bent and place one hand on your chest and the other on your abdomen, just below your ribs. Take a slow breath in through your nose, imagining the air escaping towards your lower belly. The hand on your chest should remain still while the hand on your abdomen rises. When exhaling the reverse should occur: tighten your abdominal muscles to allow air out through pursed lips and the hand on your belly should go back to the original position.

The power of the breath in exerting an influence over your emotions is evident when you experience a panic attack, asthma attack or any moment of shortness of breath, be it choking or in a claustrophobic environment. These heightened negative emotions come to the fore in people with serious lung issues like chronic obstructive pulmonary disease, where difficult breathing leads to faster, more shallow breaths and compounds anxiety and discomfort.

In taking care of your lungs, be mindful of air pollutants. Unfortunately, this is largely inescapable in modern life. Even so, there are measures you can take to ensure good air quality inside your home. Keeping it clean can minimise the accumulation of dust, while you can ensure good ventilation by periodically opening windows. Even keeping house plants is known to improve air quality by absorbing moisture (a factor in the formation of lung-unfriendly mould) and helping to regulate humidity. Other simple measures can help, like avoiding the mixing of ammonia and bleach when carrying out household chores, as the resulting gas produced can be hazardous to lung health.

[Half Page Illustration To Come]

Health Hack

As well as expelling carbon dioxide from your lungs, breathing out and giving your breath a cheeky sniff test can also help you assess your health. If you detect the following niffs, check in with a health professional:

* A sour smell can indicate acid reflux. This means bits of food are making their way back towards the throat, making it a fertile breeding ground for bacteria.

* A smell like mothballs can be a sign that you're suffering from an allergy or a cold.

* A metallic smell is often a sign of a bacterial infection in the gumline.

* Fruity-smelling breath indicates high levels of ketones in the blood. This is a sign of diabetic ketoacidosis, in which the body doesn't produce enough insulin to use as fatty acids to make energy.

* A sweet or mouldy note to your breath could be a sign of fetor hepaticus, which is an indicator of liver disease.

* Fishy breath is a sign of end-stage renal failure, in which the kidneys fail to get rid of toxic waste like urea and ammonia.

5. Failure to Load

THE SHORTCOMINGS OF THE SKELETON

YOUR BONES ARE A BIG DEAL. You'd be a mess without them. Bones are your body's infrastructure. When connected in the form of the human skeleton, thanks to the cartilage, joints and tendons that string it altogether, they're the load-bearing beams and joints that provide strength, stability and keep everything upright.

The fact that your skeleton allows you to stand on two feet is one of the reasons you are the most successful creature on earth. (Although that view depends on who you talk to.) Sometimes this same framework which nurtures, protects and supports you can also be a bony cage in which you are tortured by chronic backache, niggling neck pain and knee joints like old concrete that crumbles under pressure.

In this light, if your skeleton was a building it would be more economical and efficient to bulldoze it and build a modern replacement. While it can fail you miserably, let's figure out some architectural patch-up jobs for the critical features so the whole thing doesn't completely fall apart in your lifetime.

Close to the bone

The overall scaffolding that holds up your body, from the crown of your head to the tips of your toes, isn't just an inert substance. Your bones are very much alive. Thanks to a rich supply of blood in the thin membranous layer which covers your bones – the periosteum – they're actually a very light shade of pink, not white. You have 206 bones in your body, which do more than help you to run, jump and walk. They also protect your fragile innards, contain bone marrow and even store precious minerals like calcium and phosphorus. In order for your bones to keep protecting you, however, it's vital that you maintain them.

Human bones are like an IKEA flat pack kit. They require some building. Your bone density continually increases until your thirties. In your forties, it starts to fall as your skeleton begins to wither away and in women this process can accelerate after menopause. In your senior years, bones can fracture far more easily than they did when you were younger. So, no more wheelies over the speed bumps on your BMX.

Save yourself

You can help to maintain bone density for as long as possible with a few simple actions, and it doesn't just come down to exercise.

You've probably always been told you need to drink milk for strong bones. This is propaganda from Big Milk. The fact is most humans actually lose the ability to digest lactose shortly after birth. What's more, milk doesn't contain enough calcium to maintain your bones. If your body doesn't get enough calcium, it can leech it from your bones in order to prop up your heart and muscles – obviously this isn't ideal. Happily, other dairy products like cheese and vegetables such as kale are rich in calcium. Then we come to vitamin D, which aids the absorption of calcium from the gut, and all the more reason to soak up some rays through skin drenched in sunscreen. Before you ask . . .no, sunscreen does not 'reduce' vitamin D production. There is still roughly 3% of UV rays which can reach your skin which is more than sufficient to synthesis vitamin D. More importantly there is no such thing as a safe tan.

ON YOUR KNEES

Your knees are the workhorse of your body. These titans routinely lift the equivalent of up to six times your weight with every laborious step (even more if running!), making it the most taxed joint you own. It's designed to withstand millions of steps in your life, and yet inevitably the accumulation of stress can sometimes cause it to break down,

Walking around is great except when it hurts. The weaknesses of the knee boils down to simply anatomy and structural engineering. A hinge joint, the knee holds the bottom of your femur (thigh bone) to the top of your tibia (shin bone) by ligaments and muscle, all of which are prone to tearing and being sprained.

By comparison, the hip joint is the one that wins all the prizes for innovation. It's a ball and socket design, in which a concavity in the pelvis known as the acetabulum allows the round head of the femur to glide gracefully inside it. This makes the hip sturdy and allows a greater range of motion to accommodate easy twisting and turning. Just imagine your dance moves if your knees could do the same thing. Then again, if the knee could rotate like the hip, chances are you'd be prone to more accidents. The knee is intended to move forwards and backwards like a door hinge. If it could twist as well that would make you deeply unstable on your feet.

When you're rapidly changing direction, effectively twisting and turning, then the knee is no longer aligned with the foot. Instead, it relies on ligaments and muscles to maintain stability. Just think about that for a moment: the only things holding the two halves of your leg together when you're moving are strings and webbing. Nice job.

One such ligament, the anterior cruciate ligament (ACL), is so neglected it contains no blood vessels, and yet it has a hugely important role. It's designed to keep your femur connected to your tibia and if you tear it then only surgery can repair the damage. ACL tears are some of the most common sporting injuries we see as surgeons, in the same way that garage mechanics see a lot of cars with wheels knackered by potholes.

Save yourself

The muscles and ligaments that support the knee also rely on the quadriceps and hips for stability. Lunges and squats are simple movements to keep both the knee and hip well supported, but what of safeguarding the joint itself? This requires a sixth sense, literally . . .

Proprioception is the hidden ability you didn't know you possessed. It allows you to know the position of your joints in space – known as your spatial orientation – without looking. This is down to the fact that your joints and ligaments are saturated with nerve fibres that constantly feed back signals to your brain. Think of it as your internal body compass.

Proprioception isn't a static thing. It can be improved. Essentially, the better your body's ability to auto-calibrate or correct itself without thought, the lower your risk of injury. For example, if you're running on an uneven surface then your body is making numerous micro calculations to steady itself and limit damage to the knee. That most elite fell or mountain runners are able to make their performance seem effortless is in part due to heightened senses of proprioception, and this comes down to experience.

You can improve your proprioception with simple balance exercises. With your eyes closed, stand on one leg that is slightly bent. This forces the muscles around the knee to work harder to maintain your balance and fine-tunes your joint sense. You can turn up the difficulty by moving your head to one side, as this meddles with your inner ear balance too.

Alongside balance exercises, the more you partake in regular physical activity, the more your body and brain will instinctively know what to do and how to protect you without conscious signals from you. Ultimately, your knees will thank you.

We can rebuild it

In the UK, over 70,000 knee replacement operations take place every year. The vast majority are down to osteoarthritis. This is basically your body trying to rub your bones together to start a fire.

In a healthy human specimen, there should be a smooth gliding surface that the bones use to move around and avoid rubbing directly against each other. This is called the articular cartilage, but over time it becomes progressively thinner and worn out. The issue is that this cartilage doesn't replace itself because when it evolved to be part of your body it never assumed it would be put to work for seventy-plus years. You will use this cartilage well beyond its stated warranty period. By the time you are eighty-five, and if you've lived a reasonably active life, you could have covered 300,000 kilometres in total distance. That's almost eight times around the world. No wonder your poor cartilage gives up. Factor in excess body weight, which is the scourge of modern life, and sometimes also genetic factors, and you can see why the articular cartilage in your knees opts for early retirement. The good news is that a new knee can effectively lead to a second life. It's just sensible to take care of the original model and not wear out the tread needlessly.

Save yourself

If stress on the joint contributes to osteoarthritis then does that excuse you from hammering it with exercise like running? Before you stay on the sofa for your own good, there is evidence to suggest that slipping on your trainers and heading out for a jog can in fact stave off osteoarthritis for longer.

During a weight-bearing activity like running, the knee joint is placed under load. This helps to squeeze the cartilage like a sponge, wringing out waste and drawing in a fresh batch of nutrient-rich fluid with every step or stride. Just like most things in life, of course, moderation is key.

FEET FIRST

It's highly likely that you've spent very little of your precious time contemplating the intricacies and vagaries of your feet. The only time you might pay attention is when they get sore . . . or break.

Your foot has twenty-six individual bones. That's a total fifty-two bones in both feet. That amounts to a quarter of your skeleton. Ridiculous. Now, all those little bones, muscles and ligaments were great for your tree-dwelling ancestors, but maybe not so much now they've been repurposed for pavements. Constantly pushing off the ground means a life of plantar fasciitis, foot pains and ankle sprains.

In a perverse way, your foot woes are a small price to pay for the mobility they afford. They provide stability, the ability to move across long distances and support your contorting body as you take over the dance floor. If you did away with all those bones you would have to give up some strength, flexibility and balance, and they'd also be pressure-sensitive. On the upside, your delicate, downgraded new feet would probably put podiatrists out of business.

Until we can 3D-print new feet, you'll just have to learn to live with the sophisticated pair that connect you to the ground. With some basic care and attention, they should keep you upright before anything above it lets you down.

Save yourself

There is an argument to be made that many biomechanical foot problems can be caused by the very footwear designed to cushion and protect it. Barefoot, when your sole comes into contact with the ground, the dense receptors across your skin, tendons and ligaments relay a rich feed of information to the brain and spinal cord. This include not just data on position but also tension, force and stretch. In return, the brain provides more precise control of the muscles in your foot to adjust the joints in order to minimise impact and maximise absorption of forces to limit damage. So, why are you blunting these signals by encasing your feet in shoes? It's a hot topic in the world of running, for example, with proponents on either side making convincing cases. Clearly, there is a trade-off to be had between wanting to protect your feet and optimising foot health. Ultimately, it come down to personal choice, and the recent rise in 'minimalist' shoes goes some way towards an informed compromise. If you do decide to ditch the trainers completely, literally walk before you run. Otherwise, you risk injury by doing too much too soon.

Regardless of footwear, your feet don't demand much, even though they should. Make sure you actually bend down and cut your toenails to avoid pesky ingrown ones. As someone who has operated on a few, you do not want this. It also goes without saying you should get properly fitted shoes, both in size and width because you'll be spending most of the day in them. Ill-fitting shoes are a common culprit for corns, calluses, bunions and chronic foot pain.

In most cases some foot dryness or a few cracks here and there might not make a world of difference to the average person. If you have diabetes or a form of immune suppression, however, then that crack can become an ulcer or a wound that is painful and hard to heal. Whatever the state of your health, treat your feet like your face and keep them moisturised.

GOT BACK

Back pain is a quietly stalking assassin. It can creep up when you least expect it with devastating consequences. It's also terrible at its job because back pain rarely kills you. It just makes your life miserable.

Your spine is quite literally as the backbone of your body, and can make its presence felt in various ways, from simple aches to violent torturous spasms, scoliosis, kyphosis and searingly painful disc herniations. It even tries to shrink you every day. For such a vital role, it's incredible quite how catastrophic the spine can be in terms of engineering. We're talking about an off balance tower of delicate bones known as vertebrae, tasked with supporting a blood-filled watermelon on top. It's like trying to balance an apple stem side up. Not an easy task and one that frequently goes wrong.

In terms of achieving stability, you'd think the appropriate design for the spine would be the stiffer, straighter rod as rocked by your close relatives the chimpanzee and monkey. Instead, like one of those decisions reached by committee rather than through common sense, your spine is flexible and curvy. It's claimed these bends help you balance and walk upright, but from a physics points of view the weak spots it creates is asking for failure.

But perhaps most alarming is the fact that your body has evolved such specialised neurons in the spine that they have lost their ability to regenerate. If the spinal cord is injured the neurons can't invoke an automatic heal function, as is the case in various other parts of the body. Usually, the result is paralysis.

Save yourself

When it comes to fixing back issues, a world of misinformation and danger exists that can sometimes just make a problem worse. For all the miracle cures on offer, sometimes simple exercise is key to alleviating pain and restoring both mobility and strength.

In my opinion, spinal manipulation is not a good thing. Chiropractic-type spine and neck manipulation is not grounded in any medical science and in some cases, it can even risk serious health consequences such as vertebral artery dissection (a tearing of a vital artery which can cause strokes).

Other activities like massage, although not significantly covered by empirical evidence, are pretty harmless. In fact, this approach certainly makes sense from a pain relief perspective. It will unlikely lead to long-term changes in the back but it seems to at least improve symptoms and function in the short term. Acupuncture is poorly understood by traditional medicine, although there is evidence to suggest it seems to help – sort of. It is one of the oldest approaches to back pain and a cornerstone of traditional eastern medicine, which underpins the Chinese philosophy that disease is a result of an imbalance between yin and yang. While I am trained in traditional medicine, I was brought up in a culture with deep ties to holistic and natural remedies. So, if I suffered from back problems and nothing else worked, I would be more than happy to try acupuncture if it gave me a shot at restoring the mobility and flexibility we often take for granted.

Back pain can be a demonic force; thankfully, for the vast majority of people, it is very unlikely to be lethal. Here's my advice on when you should take back pain seriously and check in with your GP:

1. It's been troubling you for more than six weeks.

2. Your back pain is preceded by any trauma you might have been involved with like a road traffic accident.

3. The pain is severe and/or not improving or is getting even worse.

4. You have pain and weakness in both legs and/or experience an inability to pee or poo or both (an indication of nerve compression or damage).

Twists and turns

It isn't just the load that can cause problems for your spine. The basic act of movement can also cause mayhem. For example, whether you're a human, ostrich or a tiger you've got to create enough force and friction with the ground to propel yourself forward and also protect your body from the forces generated each time your feet push off. In humans, because your selfish ancestors decided to try their hand at being bipedal, all that force enters the body through a single point in your heel. It means we rely on the muscles in our lower legs to absorb much of that energy and protect our joints as it travels towards the spine. Naturally, your back is going to take some impact, and much of it can be further offset by the manner in which you move, which is called your gait.

When your heel strikes the ground, you flex your knee around 5 to 6 degrees. This allows the quads to absorb the energy. Next, as the ball of your foot pushes off the ground the quad muscle contracts, which creates the force against the ground that propels you forward. That's a lot of force coming through one contact point. So, you've adapted your gait to mitigate all that pressure with each step, which is why you swing your arms as you move. As a result, you're constantly twisting to further disperse the torsional load from your weirdo bipedal gait.

Without this twist, the reactive force from the ground would be strong enough to spin you around. The catch is that it's another major source of back problems. This is because in between each vertebral disc in your spine rests a cushion of collagen filled with a mucoprotein gel. It's a structure that's often compared to that of a jam donut. The discs allow our spine to twist and flex, and also share the load distributed through it. The trouble is that twisting millions of times over our lifetime really does a number on the discs. Sometimes the tough outer layer wears out, the jam escapes the doughnut and you earn yourself a herniated disc. Worse still, the jam can push on vital nerves, causing pain or numbness that sometimes refers (or travels) to sites from the lower back and buttocks to your feet. You can try to stave off the worst of it by strengthening your core muscles for added spinal support and stability. At the same time, you should also remember that this is a relatively small price to pay for standing upright, which is what makes us human and the number one most successful primate.

Pull yourself together

As a child, and possibly peaking in your teenage years, you will have been told to stop slouching. You may even have grown up to self-correct that tendency to let your spine sag as if you've lost the will to live. Chances are you're well aware that a good posture can reduce the risk of back and mobility issues, but it's also more nuanced than you might think.

It makes sense that constantly hunching over, staring at your phone for several hours a day, is unlikely to benefit your spine. In fact, there is even some anecdotal evidence that incidents of cervical kyphosis is on the rise, also known as 'text neck'.

Poor posture is something that is habitual and self-imposed, and it will ultimately bring you physical pain. Let's take sitting on a chair with one ankle tucked under your bum. The chair isn't forcing you into adopting a posture that will cause your spine to load unevenly. This is about you misusing the chair. You might even worsen the situation by digging your ankle in deeper in a bid to get comfortable. We're talking about shitty ergonomics. So, the solution isn't the creation of a special chair for you that accommodates one leg under a butt cheek. The answer is for you to sit in the chair correctly.

We all have our own postural quirks, of course. No doubt you try to minimise the kind of movements or resting positions that are uncomfortable, but sometimes finding ourselves ergonomically compromised can be a hazard of the job. As a surgeon, I often find myself working with sharp instruments in tight spaces and at funny angles that demand all manner of body contortions. In the case of laparoscopic surgery (a minimally invasive abdominal procedure), I need to look at a screen while using an elongated instrument skewered inside my patient's tummy. The instrument is operated by foot pedals. This means I need to ensure the correct angle and position of my hands, elbows and wrists to avoid any excessive repetitive straining. At the same time, the height of the operating table has to be comfortable for both me and my assistant. If any one of those considerations aren't carefully aligned, my patient leaves the theatre on the road to recovery while I face a path of grinding pain and a hobbling example of the overlap between bad posture triggered by postural stresses.

[Half Page Illustration To Come]

Health Hack

Here's a health hack to save you time and energy. There's a great deal to be said for working out and getting the most out of your body, but the fact is there are limits. The average human body calls upon roughly 60 per cent of muscle mass at peak exertion; a professional athlete might crank that up to 80 per cent, but there's a reason why we keep the rest in reserve.

If you had access to 100 per cent muscle strength, it wouldn't end well. You might appear to have superhuman strength compared to ordinary mortals, but your muscles would tear off the bone, breaking them in the process and shredding ligaments and tendons. So, the next time you hit the gym, chill just a little bit.

6. Eyes Up

PARTIAL ADVENTURES
IN SIGHT

THEY'VE BEEN THE SUBJECT OF POETRY and philosophy for centuries, and yet essentially we're talking about two balls of salted jelly. I don't want to merely cover mechanistic details about how the eyes work (by converting light signals to electrical code in the brain) but look at more practical aspects about how you can offset the inevitable decline in your visual health over time. With the facts to hand, you might even find ways to reinforce your sight abilities. Oddly enough, you could even leverage it to optimise other aspects of your health further afield from the eye, such as your physical and even mental health.

Vision on

Your eyes are as great as they are terrible. In fact, an argument could be made for the case that all humans are basically blind, even those with supposedly perfect vision. The fact is we are blind to approximately 99.997 per cent of the world. The full rainbow of radiation, the electromagnetic spectrum, is probably a beautiful thing but you'll never see it because only a fraction of this is accessible to the human eye: a measly 0.0035 per cent known as visible light. You continue your ordinary life oblivious to the hidden world around you.

Evolution has bound us to these limitations because realistically we don't need X-ray or infrared vision to dodge predators or find a suitable mate. Bees and butterflies, on the other hand, do need UV radiation to identify special patterns on flowers, while snakes require infrared vision to hunt their warm-blooded victims. We are all in some way slaves to our evolutionary destinies and roles in this simulation.

Wiping the tapes

The misery of the eye doesn't end there. In fact, it is so appalling in construct that the brain has to cover for it and lie to you. Even now, while reading this page, you are going blind momentarily. This quirk is known as saccadic masking, a fancy term for the brain doing a cover-up job for your shoddy ability to see and deleting your eyes' incriminating CCTV footage. This is because every time your eyes move or shift, such as when reading the page of a book, it pieces together a series of still images. Many of these are blurred as the eyes move, and so the brain dispatches those to the cutting room floor to at least pretend that what you're looking at is rendered smooth and cinematic.

The rapid movements your eye makes when shifting in gaze is called a saccade. Conversely, the place where your eye comes to rest is known as a fixation point. When you look between fixation points, the blurred images that the brain deletes along the way are in fact moments of blindness. Just in case you cotton on to the deceit, your brain even blocks your conscious mind from registering it. Who can you trust, eh?

The upside down

Once upon a time (blame the Ancient Greeks for this one), we used to think that we saw the world thanks to light that beamed from our eyes to illuminate the objects we see. This was known as emission theory and it dominated our understanding of vision for centuries.

Thankfully, we saw sense in the sixteenth century and evolved our understanding of eye mechanics. This is when we recognised that the eye is a conduit of sorts with the retina acting as a receptor of light. As it hits the cornea, light is refracted (or bent) by the lens to form an image on the retina at the back of the eye. This is where it gets strange. You receive a crystal clear image but it's upside down, because the process of refraction via a convex lens causes images to be inverted. To right this wrong, your brain has to pick up the pieces and flip the image to make it right-side-up. If you don't believe how terrible your eyes are when it comes to one simple task, close your eyelids and gently press the bottom left of your eyeball. In doing so, you should notice a dark spot appear in the top right corner, thus proving the flipping image has been flipped.

It's worth noting that this flipping act isn't something we're born to perform. It has to be learned by the brain. It's believed that in the first few days of life, babies still see the world upside down. Not good. So, if a newborn cries in fear when glancing at your face, it may not be your challenging visage that spikes fear into its heart but the fact that your smile has yet to be converted from a frown.

Wretched retinas

You have to understand that evolution isn't down to a neurosurgeon using microsurgical techniques to shape the way humans were created. Evolution is ham-handed, messy, disorganised but quirky, and this is evident in the construction of your eyes. Once the process began, there was no going back. Mistakes were piled on top of mistakes and covered over time by shortcuts and diversions so you weren't left floundering in the dark.

To provide some rose-tinted nostalgia, or simply to stir up bad memories, it's worth thinking back to that school biology science lesson where you most likely saw a sectional anatomical illustration of the eye detailing various internal structures. The first important structure to note here is the retina: the switchboard of the eye that receives incoming communication (in the form of light) and relays it to the brain for processing.

In fact, your retina is technically part of your brain, the only part of it which sits on the outside world, beyond the protection of the cranial vault. So you basically have two pieces of brain tissue that got purposely squeezed out during embryonic development and plopped inside two eye sockets.

A more detailed close-up of the retina reveals its individual layers. Here, the rods and cones (light-sensitive cells known as photoreceptors) are only reached after light travels through the entire gamut of cell layers and neurons to reach them. Generally speaking, rods cells handle light and come into their own at night, while the cones bring colour into the mix. While both rods and cones are fit for purpose, a design flaw lies in the fact that the retina housing them appears to be facing inwards rather than outwards. In 2015, a group of scientists reached the conclusion that this arrangement might serve to prevent us from being overwhelmed – or blinded – by light, but it still strikes me as odd that photons of light are

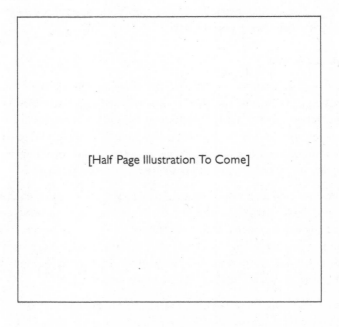

[Half Page Illustration To Come]

forced to take the long route around the entire 'camera cell' to hit the receiving side. Perhaps this comes down to the fact that your eyes evolved as an outgrowth of the brain rather than a folding in of the outer skin of your face.

Due to this haphazard arrangement, and the fact the nerve fibres from the rods and cones are required to reach a confluence to join the optic nerve on a journey back to the brain, this leaves you with an unfortunate predicament. Basically, you have a hole in the front-facing (but technically the back) side of the retina to allow the optic nerve to traverse, which presents itself through your vision as an accidental blind spot. Helpfully, or sneakily depending on your opinion, the brain compensates by filling in the blanks with existing stock footage from its photo library. It also factors in compensatory mechanisms from each eye, so they help one another out. Most of the time we don't perceive the existence of such blind spots, and it doesn't bear a great compromise to our visual function. Even so, if our retinas were fitted in reverse (or indeed the most efficient, or *correct* way), you wouldn't have this problem at all.

In order to make up for the fact that the blind spot lacks photoreceptors, the human eye also has a sweet spot called the macula. This is a part of the retina that is densely packed with rods and cones for fine, detailed vision. Further within the macula is another area called the fovea centralis, which is reserved exclusively for a high density of cones. This eggs-in-one-basket approach is quite risky because it makes you so reliant on the macula for detailed vision. It means any problems with that small area will have a major impact on your ability to see clearly, because sadly the remainder of your retina is not high-powered enough due to a diffuse spread of rods and cones. As it turns out, macular degeneration is the most common cause of blindness. You can blame funky anatomy for this Achilles eye heel.

Who can you trust?

What you see is a lie. This might sound like an Orwellian statement, but the fact that the rods and cones of the retina are good at different things means without your brain to remix things your vision would be a mess. At the periphery of your vision, you're mostly fitted with rod cells. These see in black and white and are pretty poor at clarity compared to the fine detail you can detect from the densely clustered, cone-dominated centre. Yet despite this odd arrangement, you perceive a full colour image seemingly in all parts of your eye. Essentially, the lack of colour vision and fine detail from the edges is compensated by the brain's extrapolation of stored information. It calls upon material in this library to stitch together assumptive data based on past experiences known as 'unconscious inference'.

With this in mind, everything you can see at this very moment is simply guesswork. It's a concept that gives me existential panic, and so I hope it does the same for you because misery shared is misery halved. Let's say you look at a red apple. The colour-capable cone cells in your eye are in fact formulating a pattern of electrical code and data points based on the wavelength of light reflected off the apple to allow you to perceive the red colour. So, is the apple actually red? Yes and no. There is no red light that enters your eye. Instead, your brain compares the wavelengths of light reflecting off the red apple to the other wavelengths around that object. You are simply perceiving a pattern of electricity – a comparison of different electrical signals – and what you are seeing is a translation of signals. So, it might be more appropriate to say you see with your brain and gather information with your eyes.

Red mist

It isn't just the backwards arrangement of photoceptors which is odd, nor the nerve plugged into that valuable real estate at the front of your eye. Just to add to the compromised design, the blood vessels that supply the retina sits on the world-facing side and so comes between the light and photo receptive layer. Typically, this doesn't cause too much carnage, although it does contribute to the blind spot and limit the amount of light that reaches the rods and cones. More significantly, however, it increases the risk of eye diseases.

It's a fact that the majority of people who suffer with diabetes will also experience diabetic retinopathy, that is the slow destruction of the retina. In response to chronic reduced blood oxygen availability, caused by the disease, the retina responds by nudging the vessels to proliferate in a desperate plea to boost supply. As they sit in front of the retina, the increase just serves to worsen vision all the more. Once again, all this nonsense could have been avoided if your eyes just had their retinal placement rejigged. Sadly, it's too late for us to do anything about that.

Another consequence of nature not giving us attractive, squid-like eyes but a bloody awful 'backward' retina is the increased susceptibility to retinal detachment. In cephalopod eyes, the axons of photoreceptor cells (long pole-like bodies) anchor the retina to the layers underneath. In human eyes, the retina can become detached from the pigmented layer underneath. This detached piece of retina can subsequently lose its bloody supply and cause blindness in the affected segment.

Blocked eyeballs

Moving away from mob lynching your retina for a moment, let's take a look at some poor eye construction that can cause anarchy. You might have heard of a condition called glaucoma, which is the result of an increased intra-ocular pressure, specifically in the anterior chamber of the eye. The chamber is filled with clear fluid called aqueous humour, and yet what I'm about to tell you is anything but laughable. This liquid is usually drained through pipework called the trabecular meshwork. Unfortunately, sloppy plumbing and the location of these drainage pipes, between the iris and cornea, means they are susceptible to becoming blocked. If this aqueous humour builds up and raises the eye pressure it can damage the optic nerve resulting in blindness. If we're handing out review stars here, aim low. Would not recommend.

Ripped vision

Moving from inner furnishing to external fittings, we need to have a word about your eye muscles. Known as extraocular muscles you have six in total: the lateral, medial, superior, inferior rectus, inferior and superior oblique. Strictly speaking, that's three too many. If you imagine your eye to be a sphere, from a physics viewpoint you could easily manage with three muscles to move it in all directions. Going to six might sound like the kind of boast that applies to the number of blades on the latest razor, and indeed just like shaving technology you really don't need that many. Ultimately, it increases the chances of something going wrong, which can significantly impair your vision.

Crashing the car

By comparison, the visual mechanics of your eyes are somewhat basic compared to the computational tasks like depth perception. This literally requires the brain to do on-the-spot calculus and trigonometry to make sense of what limited data the eye provides. This takes the form of a two-dimensional image of the world, which the brain then renders into three dimensions based on your memory and past experiences. On a very basic level, it knows that objects seem to diminish in size with distance and can remind us that things are stationary as you pass them by even though they cross our field of vision. Without processing and interpreting this ocular information, you wouldn't last a minute behind the wheel of a car without ending up in a ditch.

We live in a world that champions the eyes for allowing us to process images, shapes, colours and movement, but actually their job is really just as emissaries of the brain. The most primal and basic function of the eye is to help us detect light levels to communicate the time of day to the mothership inside the cranium. This function comes about thanks to one of the most ancient of cells called the melanopsin ganglion cells, a special type of neuron that connects the retina to the brain. It even contains its own photoreceptors and photopigment, melanopsin. Interestingly the melanopsin pigment is also found in the skin of amphibians like frogs. This allows them to alter skin colour in response to light, which is a trick sadly denied to the likes of you. The melanopsin retinal ganglion cells perform mainly non-image-forming visual functions like regulating sleep–wake cycles, mood, cognition, the release of various hormones and metabolic rate. As long as you have a retina, even if you have compromised vision, these cells will be present to help govern the non-image functions.

Eyes and shine

On an evolutionary note, human eyeballs are growing longer and more pear-shaped. This results in the cornea becoming overly curved so light is focused in front of the retina instead of on the retina, which means that close objects seem clear but distant ones become blurry. The primary culprits are thought to be more exposure to screens and less exposure to natural light in the daytime, which is thought to have protective benefits against myopia (or nearsightedness). It's a condition that can have serious consequences, such as an increased risk of long-term glaucoma and macular degeneration. This is a slow decay of the macula in the middle of the retina, ultimately culminating in loss of direct vision.

Save yourself

From a practical standpoint, there are measures you can take to protect your eyes and reduce the risk of myopia and other ocular issues. If you spend a lot of time in front of a screen (which is likely to be most people), then adopt the 20/20/20 rule. Every 20 minutes, take a break from the screen and look at a distant object at least 20 feet away for up to 20 seconds. This allows the eyes to relax and turn the focus off momentarily. It's also good to get away from the screen, right? So why not pop outside and dose up on natural light?

Focusing the eyes and mind

Every time you look at something, whether far or near, your eye dynamically adjusts where the reflected light lands by transforming the shape of the lens. This process is known as accommodation and it has a greater impact than just allowing us to see clearly up close and at a distance. It also has relevance to cognitive focus and mental relaxation.

Each time your lens changes shape, it is at the behest of a troupe of tiny helpers called ciliary muscles. At the same time, the iris and its sphincter muscles adjust the amount of light entering the lens. So, when you view something in the distance, the lens relaxes and flattens; this relaxation in turns provides you and your eyes with a relaxing effect when looking at a panoramic view. By contrast, focusing on an object nearby requires more effort from the intricate muscles around the lens. Even the iris is required to put in some effort to make the lens contract and become fatter. This focuses light on to the retina to the actual extraocular muscles that move the eyeball within its socket.

The relevance of this seemingly obscure crumb of anatomy might not be immediately apparent, but then nowadays we spend a significant chunk of our days looking at objects close to our faces. Peering at phones, documents and computer screens isn't allowing the eye lenses to relax and for the muscles to take a break. This is a fast track to eye pain, which might ultimately contribute to headaches.

Save yourself

Optic flow is a concept that refers to the sensation of perceiving your surroundings moving in relation to your own body moving, like the trees moving past you when you cycle through a forest. You can achieve this state of optic flow through any self-generated movement like cycling, running, hiking and even swimming. Why is optic flow good for us? Your visual system is also part of your autonomic nervous system, which includes the sympathetic nervous system. This is the body's fight-or-flight control unit. When facing an imminent lion attack, or just everyday stress, it can dilate your pupils to give you a narrow field of focus.

We also have to consider the parasympathetic nervous system here. This is in charge of rest and digestion. It's the system that helps us to relax. On a visual level, it constricts your pupils and widens your field of focus. This function is optimised in states of optic flow, which can be achieved by viewing a panorama while moving through it. You can achieve optic flow by walking indoors, but it's a more rewarding, holistic experience when you head outside and take in your surroundings.

Super vision

Even though your eye can be found wanting on more than one occasion, its ability to adapt under pressure is interesting if slightly confusing. Our vision underwater is a case in point. It blurs because the surrounding water has the same density as the water contained by the outer cornea, which means we lose some refractive power. It might sound like something you just have to live with, but there is a precedent to suggest you simply need to try harder. The Moken people are a nomadic, sea-loving tribe that live in the archipelagos of the Andaman Sea. The children spend their days diving underwater scouting for food. Incredibly, they are able to see underwater with perfect clarity and without the stinging burn associated with salt-infused eyes.

It's believed that over time, and with frequent exposure to swimming underwater with their eyes open, the Moken people have developed lenses that can change shape to maintain their refractive power, as well as pupils that contract to increase their depth of field. What is still a mystery, however, is how their eyes remain immune to the burning of seawater. Tough kids, I guess.

Don't stare at the su ...

Your eye socket dumplings are precious. Not only can they sting madly in seawater, but they're also prone to damage from something 93 million miles away. Hopefully, you learned from an early age that staring at the sun is a bad idea. To understand why, imagine a child using a magnifying glass to fry some ants (assuming the child is malevolent). While the glass can focus the sun rays on to a single point to amplify the energy, the lens contained within your eye is about four times the strength. It's capable of burning holes through a sheet of paper, so just think of what can happen to your retina should you be foolish enough to face the fiery orb.

In some cases, people can develop such severe damage to their vision that there's a condition named after it. Solar retinopathy arises due to permanent damage to the part of your retina that provides you with the most detailed vision, the fovea centralis. As a result, sufferers have to live with blurry vision or a big dark spot in their field of view, plus a whole heap of regret.

What happens when you rub your eyes?

Some of what I've revealed about your eyes might sound downright ridiculous. You might even rub yours in disbelief, but that's exactly what you should never do unless you're aiming to give them a horrifying DIY makeover and literally change their shape.

When you manhandle your eyeballs with your fingertips or knuckles, you're literally squishing them inside your eye sockets and deforming them ever so slightly. That's not even the worst part. It doesn't just sound bad, it literally harms your eyeball. In fact, there is evidence to suggest that constantly rubbing your eyeballs could be a cause of keratoconus. This is a condition in which the cornea bulges out and your eyeball literally changes shape due to excessive eye rubbing.

Worst psychedelic trip ever

If you've ever squished your eyes then chances are you've also experienced the 'in-head' display of swirls, colours and flashes known as phosphenes. This free psychedelic show is the result of your poor confused eye perceiving light when there is none.

The retinal ganglion cells which interpret light are easily tricked. In short, they can be activated through the application of pressure. If you gently press into your eye now, the ganglion cells are fooled into firing off information to your brain in the same way they would be if stimulated via light. They cannot physically tell the difference between light and pressure information and so translate it in the same way to the visual cortex of your brain. As a result, you perceive the kind of light show that might dazzle as a careful one off. Just be aware that repeatedly poking your eyes for a performance could cause backstage problems.

Warning signs

When you're staring at something uniform or bright, like the sky or a white sheet of paper, chances are you'll see 'eye floaters'. These are random, worm-like or fuzzy moving structures in your field of vision. Their medical name is muscae volitantes, or 'flying flies', but fear not, your eyes haven' been invaded by parasitic creatures. These tiny objects are in fact random clumps of protein such as detached tissue fragments or even red blood cells. They can cast a shadow on your retina as they swim through the vitreous humour (the jelly-like substance that keeps the shape of your eye) and pass through the light that enters your eye.

While seeing these things can be normal, and nothing to worry about, if you do notice a sudden increase in the amount of these floaters – often accompanied by a sensation of sudden flashing light – then I'd advise you to get seen by an eye doctor immediately. It can be a symptom of something known as retinal detachment, in which the retina tears away and leads to loss of vision.

Face lungs

I've often thought of the eyeballs as the lungs of the face. Your corneas don't have any blood supply, in fact they're the only part of the human body to survive without it. Instead, it gets its fill of oxygen directly from the air. So, when you wear contacts, the oxygen supply to your cornea reduces slightly. This further tanks when you close your eyes to sleep. This is why sleeping with your contacts in place is a short-sighted idea on several levels. The low oxygen environment in the eyeballs of sleeping contact lens wearers is enough to cause the cornea to swell up. This results in gaps forming between the superficial cells of your eye that can attract bacteria. Allowing your eyeball to become a petri dish overnight makes any eye infection a source for concern. Why? Because your eye is an immune-privileged site, which means it doesn't quite have the same level of protection as other places in your body. This makes some sense: if your immune system caused eye inflammation every time something irritated your eye, as you'd be living with frequently compromised vision.

Any contact lens wearer who does go through the night knows there is nothing worse than peeling one off your eye once you wake up. It risks further irritation and even damage to the cornea

Night vision

In a bid to see in the dark, back when I was very young, I ate an entire bag of carrots for a week. The transformative effects went no further than turning me orange, and yet science suggests I wasn't the dumb kid my parents perceived me to be. Carrots are naturally rich in vitamin A (beta-carotene), which is excellent for maintaining eye health. In fact, vitamin A is a precursor of rhodopsin or 'rods', the photopigment in the retina that predominantly helps with night vision. It can even reverse night blindness in those with vitamin A deficiency. Yes, I fell for the myth that it would help me to see in the dark, but to be fair I wasn't the first.

At the beginning of the Second World War, the UK quickly – and secretly – developed proficiency in radar technology. Much to the bewilderment of German tacticians, it meant the RAF were able to shoot down a large number of enemy planes at night. Keen to protect their advantage, the British High Command fed newspapers with the story that their pilots had better night vision because they ate carrots. The ruse was such a great success that it didn't just fool the Germans but also the British public. Given the proven health benefits, the government even launched a 'Doctor Carrot' campaign and made these super-powered vegetables exempt from war rations to encourage their consumption.

(To return to the statement I casually dropped in a moment ago, did I really turn a shade of orange? It might sound like a myth but is in fact true. If you eat a high volume of carrots, or anything high in beta-carotene like pumpkins or oranges, this pigment can also turn your skin the same colour. Thankfully, I saw a full reversal of my Oompa Loompa complexion after my parents restored my carrot intake to a sensible level.)

Turn the dark up

With so many potential ocular deficits, there is always a chance that you could lose your vision at some stage. Without a doubt, the ability to see is one of the most important senses through which you can interact and perceive the world. Blindness can have devastating consequences, from increased social isolation to a susceptibility to mental health issues like depression. In some cases, however, the deficiency of one sense can amplify others. It can even lead to the emergence of extraordinary hidden superpowers, as we'll discover when we turn our attention to the ears in the following chapter.

[Half Page Illustration To Come]

Health Hack

A pair of sharp eyes could save you money when it comes to shopping for fresh produce. We know that fruit such as raspberries and blueberries are rich in antioxidants like polyphenols (protecting against heart disease and cancers), but it's worth checking the label for the country of origin before you buy.

Why? Because fuelling the demand for fruit out of season – that has often been imported from around the world – not only drives up the price but also increases you carbon footprint.

Instead, check out their frozen counterparts, which contain the same (if not higher) levels of polyphenols as they're harvested, packaged and cooled when fresh. They're also cheaper, more environmentally friendly, and you can eat them all year round.

7. All Ears

A HIKE AROUND HEARING

THE FACT THAT YOUR EARS CONSPIRE with your brain to make sense of tiny little changes in airwaves is a remarkable feat of biology. The technical term for those flappy things attached to each side of your head is auricle or pinnae (which means fin or wing in Latin). The outer part of your ear is made from cartilage and is optimised for sound capture. In fact, we still contain tiny vestigial muscles that our ancestors used to use to move their ears in response to sound. A freakish few are still able to make them swivel, which is a sight to behold.

Our perception of sound occurs when vibrations in the air, also known as sound waves, enter our ear. Those you can hear are typically limited to frequencies between 20Hz and 20,000HZ. Frequencies of sound below this are known as infrasound, and while you might not 'hear' them using your limited ears, your brain receives them via vibrations from the skull, skin and bones that make up your jaw and face. Despite being one of the smallest parts of your body, your ears are involved in more than just your sense of hearing. They also coordinate your balance and posture, which is known as vestibular function. Nowhere else in the human body are so many different functional elements so densely packed in a such a confined bony space.

A world in your ear

The three regions of the ear – outer, middle and inner ear – all have distinct but equally important roles to play. The outer and middle ear regions are primarily concerned with the relaying of sound to the inner ear. The inner ear houses a shell-like structure known as the cochlea, which essentially acts as a transducer to convert sound energy into electrical energy. The inner ear also contains the vestibular apparatus: three semicircular ducts and two chambers that contain the receptors which govern our balance and coordination.

The ear is one of those subjects I never really paid much heed to at medical school. At best it's a C-rated organ (otolaryngologists reading or listening to this are no doubt punching the air in frustration right now) – but I recognise it's still a fascinatingly strange organ. To illustrate its oddness, up to 70 per cent of people's ears make noises known as otoacoustic emissions. It's just a normal function of the cochlea, and though the sound may not be something you hear it can influence animals in your environment. So, it's like you're a dolphin now.

The beat of the drum

The sounds that get captured by your ears eventually reach the tympanic membrane or eardrum; it truly is as simple as the skin of a drum. On the inside of the eardrum are three tiny bones shaped like a hammer: the malleus, incus and stapes. Every time sound enters your ear, the membrane of your eardrum can move back and forth and cause the bones to tap the cochlea. Here's where it gets slightly crazy; the cochlea contains little hair cells – nothing to do with the hairs on your head – rather they just look like hairs under the microscope. Their role is to move in response to a beat from the malleus, incus and stapes bones and send signals to the brain. The intricate snail-shaped organisation of the cochlea is essential, not just for hearing but in discriminating different frequencies of sound. It's incredibly intricate, and vulnerable to abuse when you crank your speakers to eleven on the dial.

The haircut you didn't want

You are born with around 16,000 hair cells in your cochlea. You can sustain damage to around half of these hair cells before you notice significant changes to your hearing. By then, it will be too late to do anything about it.

You might have noticed that if you've ever been at a music concert or a sporting event, the moment you return to a quieter venue your hearing seems a bit dulled and you struggle to hear low volume sounds. This is normal because your hair cells are like blades of grass. They bend more in response to louder noises but usually return to their usual shape after a period of time. However, prolonged exposure to a loud sound can irreversibly damage the hair cells, thus resulting in gradual hearing loss.

What's too loud I hear you say? It's difficult to give an exhaustive list of things, but if you have to shout to have a conversation over the noise, your ears ring afterwards or things seem muffled after exposure then it's probably too much.

Your smartphone typically has a maximum volume of around 102 decibels. This means that even just listening to a few songs at full blast can damage your hearing. Let me be clear, there is no way to reverse damage caused to your vulnerable inner ear. These hairs do not repair themselves or grow back. It is strange that we are bestowed something so delicate and fragile that can be lost for the rest of our lives just by listening to your favourite song too loudly. We could see it as Mother Nature at her most cruel, or a constant reminder that life is precious.

Save yourself

As a general rule, in order to minimise hearing damage related to headphone use, aim to limit yourself to 60 minutes of music at around 60 per cent volume. Then take a break for 15 minutes or so. Personally, I always use over-ear headphones rather than in-ear buds as sound is applied in a less direct manner to the tympanic membrane (the eardrum).

It's also worth investing in noise-cancelling headphones. These cut out background sounds without you having to raise the volume.

Are you receiving?

Our traditional five senses each have unique receptors: photoreceptors for eyesight, olfactory receptors for smelling, taste receptors for taste and mechanoreceptors for touching. Then there's hearing, which doesn't have a specific receptor. Instead, it uses the same mechanoreceptor that our skin uses to detect touch. Of course, it works a little differently because the hair cells in which those receptors exist detect movement and not sound waves. So, it's basically just a touch receptor repurposed as a 'hearing' receptor, and works in such a finely tuned fashion that it allows us to interpret millions of sounds. You could say that talking is basically someone softly touching your ears, but I suspect that might stop you from sleeping at night.

Although your ears can detect millions of sounds, it's just a fraction of what exists in the world around you. In fact, the evolutionary limitations of your ears and auditory system might even explain some audible paranormal phenomena.

The ghosts in your ears

In the early 1980s, British engineer Vic Tandy was working late at night in his lab in Warwickshire. As the night wore on, he began to feel an intense sense of impending doom. Then, in his peripheral vision, Tandy caught sight of a grey figure stooping against the white laboratory wall. He swung around to face it, but the figure was gone.

As it happened, Tandy's colleagues had warned him about the lab before, but Tandy – sceptic that he was – refused to believe that the building was haunted by something supernatural. 'There has to be a scientific explanation,' he thought, and it turns out he was right. The culprit was the lab's newly installed extractor fan that hummed at a rate of 18.9 Hz.

The frequency of 18.9 Hz is just below the range of human hearing, which is 20 to 20,000 Hz. Now, that's a decent range, but there's still a lot of sound we can't hear. For example, elephants have a smaller range of hearing than we do, but their slightly lower frequency range means they can hear sounds that we can't, like the movement of clouds or the ghostly rumbling of an extractor fan. Then there are all manner of creatures like bats who can hear above 20,000 Hz. Who knows what's going on up there? In fact, its recently been discovered that when plants are distressed they actually scream and emit sounds at a frequency between 20,000 Hz and 100,000 Hz. In this view, maybe ghosts just communicate using high-frequency squeaks? It would make a lot of sense.

Anyway, back to Tandy's lab. How can something we can't even hear cause so much drama? Well, interestingly, sound at this frequency has been shown to cause feelings of anxiety, dizziness, and disorientation. They often use it in horror movie soundtracks to add that extra coat of creepiness. And these low-frequency sounds don't just make you *feel* on edge: they can also interfere with the vibrations of your eyeballs (yup, your eyeballs are constantly vibrating like little spherical jellies). This causes your eyes to see things that aren't actually there. Everything from wind turbines to rumbling fridges can cause these low-frequency sound waves. As most of us don't carry audio gauges with us everywhere we go, it's hard to know just how many hauntings are actually caused by a wobbly washing machine or trembling toaster.

A hidden superpower

When we locate the position of a noise in the real world we typically use a combination of sight and sound to pinpoint the source. However, blind people, despite being deprived of one sense, seem to outperform sighted individuals in their sense of hearing. Some even develop what you could consider to be a hidden superpower: echolocation or sonar.

When a person loses their vision, their brain undergoes rewiring and reorganisation. The visual cortex starts becoming more receptive to other sensory information since it no longer receives visual input. In essence, a larger brain processing output is now assigned to things like hearing, taste, touch and smell.

This reorganisation can culminate in the development of echolocation. This describes the use of clicks – such as by the mouth – to listen for echoes off surrounding objects in the environment in order to map the world. In fact, studies have even shown bursts of activity within the visual cortex in blind people who use echolocation.

Secret ear passages

It isn't just noise that can unsettle your delicate hearing. Pressure can also cause problems in the form of something called barotrauma. This is the uncomfortable 'blocked ears' sensation you can experience as a flight passenger at take-off or landing. Ear barotrauma occurs because the air pressure between the middle ear and the environment is unbalanced. In severe cases it can extend from being an annoyance to causing headaches, dizziness and even nausea.

A simple trick to equalise the pressure involves yawning. In this case, it isn't a sign of fatigue or laziness but a skill to be prized to save your ears from the stresses of the world. When you yawn or chew on some gum, you activate a muscle in the head, just behind the mouth cavity, called the tensor veli palatini. This tenses the soft palate, producing a cascade of effects that culminates in the opening of the eustachian tubes (connecting the nasal/sinus cavity with the middle ear), which can serve as a pressure regulation pipe. You might even be able to do this on command without having to yawn; these special few are known as ear clickers.

Q-tips

Sometimes the mysterious passages in our hearing holes become clogged with earwax. Besides causing your ears to stink and impairing hearing, it's actually performing a crucial role. Earwax acts as a physical barrier to germs, dirt, dust and various nefarious pathogens that try to storm the landing sites of your ears. However, this sticky ally can also turn on us. If earwax accumulates, it reduces the ability of the eardrum to vibrate effectively and generally ruins the acoustics of your ear architecture.

An excessive build-up of earwax can also lead to balance issues and even dizziness. This is because you are dependent on equilibrium being maintained between the pressure in the eustachian tubes and the outside world.

No doubt there have been times when you dunked a cotton-tipped swab (or Q-tip) into these long dark passages to scrape out the gunk. This might seem like the smart move, but it is in fact foolish and fraught with danger. Due to the narrow diameter of your lughole, prodding it with a swab is likely to jam earwax deeper into the cavity – preventing new wax from pushing out the old stuff. In notable cases, people have even accidentally perforated their eardrum by swabbing. Like most of your body's orifices, your ears weren't built to accommodate penetration from foreign objects. For the most part, it's a one-way system. Taking into account the various air pressure, ventilation and plumbing balances going on inside your ear, it's kind of obvious that thrusting a stick into it is only likely to make an existing problem worse. Thanks to the fluid-like nature of your earwax, you should think of it as a self-cleaning system.

Should you be tempted to insert things into your ears, not just to relieve an itch or unplug some earwax, but in seeking the mystic eargasm, please reconsider your life choices. The tickling sensation returned by your sensitive ear cavity might be pleasurable, but could give rise to infection.

There is another odd consequence of rummaging around in your ear that further highlights the peculiar and unnecessary designs your body takes; an automatic coughing reflex. The Arnold ear-coughing reflex, unsurprisingly named after Friedrich Arnold, the nineteenth-century German scientist who discovered it, is unusual to say the least. The cough serves no particular purpose, but arises due to its connection with the vagus nerve on its long pilgrimage from your brain to your intestines. Along the way, the nerve flirts with the top of the ear. The segment which enters the ear canal is called the Arnold nerve and is involved with the touch sensation. So, any unusual culprits found trespassing in the ear canal – be it an insect or a stray Q-tip – stimulates the main superhighway of the nerve as it travels through your neck. Even though it's a certified biological glitch, your brain doesn't value your ear highly enough to trust it, assumes the source of the irritation is coming from the throat, and fires up a cough reflex in a misguided quest to remove the offending irritant.

Rock and roll

Believe it or not, your balance is controlled by a specific component within your ears. Right next to your spiral snail-shaped cochlea, which converts sound into electrical signals, lie the semicircular canals. These are basically Hula Hoops filled with marbles that shift inside them as you move.

You have three semicircular canals in total. One is positioned vertically, the second positioned at a 45-degree angle and the last tilted at 90 degrees. As your head turns in a particular way, the marbles within the hoops roll according to the speed, direction and plane of head movement. These marbles should more accurately be called stones or otoliths. You have ear rocks. Don't ask me why the body is obsessed with rocks in all body cavities, from urine pipes to salivary pipes, but these ones are actually helpful. These ear stones are primarily built from calcium. When they move inside the hoops they can deflect microscopic hair cells that detect direction. Ultimately, your entire balance system depends on rocks moving in your ears like mini landslides, and this figures out your position in space.

Save yourself

Here's an experiment to improve your ability to regulate those rocks and improve your sense of balance. Stand on one leg, lift up the other leg and stare off into the distance. Now shut your eyes. You should feel wobbly, which is known as postural sway, because your vestibular system also relies on visual input to maintain positional balance. There is an inbuilt symbiotic relationship, in fact, in which the vestibular system tells your eyes where to move and the position of your eyes tells your balance system how to function.

Now here's the fun bit, you can actually optimise your sense of balance by shaping up your vestibular system. Begin by standing on one leg once more, but this time keep your eyes open. Look a short distance away but then keep extending your vision progressively into the distance. Next, while maintaining control of your focus as well as your balance, bring your vision back to a point closer to you. This type of vestibular training, which incorporates changing visual information, helps to coordinate the cerebellum (the mini brain at the back of your head), semicircular canals and the eyes to improve your sense of balance.

We might think of balance in terms of stillness and poise, but it's rarely static. In fact, most of your day-to-day life is about being dynamic, from walking to running or nimbly side-stepping that puddle before a car ploughs through it. So, for a few minutes each day, if you want to enhance your balancing abilities then adopt a one-legged static hold and combine it with changes in your visual environment. You can even challenge yourself further in this position by making adjustments to your body posture.

Seasickness made simple

With your eyes open, move your head very slowly to the right. Then repeat the move but do so quickly. You probably noticed it's more uncomfortable to move your head slowly. This is because the stones in the hula hoop don't pick up enough momentum to move. Instead, your eyes have to flit from one position to the next as your head moves. As a result, moving at a snail's pace can be disruptive to the balance and visual system.

When it comes to explaining why you feel sick at sea, think of those small movements magnified. As the vessel rolls slowly over wave after wave, your ear stones respond in kind, and yet your immediate surroundings (i.e. the fixtures and fittings) appear static to your eyes. As a result, a mismatch occurs between your visual and balance inputs and you begin to wish that death was an option to the kind of nausea that can consume you.

Do you hear that noise?

Your ears can be so problematic they can drive some poor souls to the point of insanity by creating non-existent noises. One commonplace example is tinnitus. A person usually experiences tinnitus as an internal buzzing, whistling tone or ringing in the ears.

While the cause of tinnitus remains somewhat mysterious, and a reflection of the complexity in the relationship between the brain and hearing, it can be a constant, internally generated intrusion. Tinnitus isn't physically harmful but can be associated with an underlying condition like head trauma, age-related hearing loss and even earwax build up. Psychologically, however, the condition can have particularly insidious consequences for your health. It's unsurprising to learn that a persistent, loud but ultimately non-existent noise can cause sufferers stress, poor sleep, difficulty concentrating, irritability and even anxiety.

[Half Page Illustration To Come]

Health Hack

You might have heard that plants thrive when you pee on them, and then chosen to be selectively deaf. The fact is there's nothing your gladioli like more than a golden shower.

* Strictly speaking, aim to pee on the soil rather than the plants. This is because urine contains a good ratio of nitrogen, phosphorus and potassium. When watered down, it's effectively an elixir of life that can be absorbed at the root.

* What's more, uric acid in wee can speed up the decomposition of compost. In this view, it's a valuable resource for every corner of your garden, and one you should deploy as a free resource to help it thrive.

8. Hold Your Nose

THE HELL OF SMELL

YOUR NOSE IS A DESIGN DISASTER. Like any pipe, it gets blocked, springs leaks and requires regular clearing. It also bleeds, discharges super-fast jets of sneeze spray and grows random tufts of annoying hair. Your brain hates your nose so much that it tricks you into pretending it isn't there. This is known as inattentional blindness, in which you fail to perceive something that is literally right in front of you. Only now that I've mentioned it you probably can't stop noticing your nose. Has it always looked like that?

Whether you're embarrassed by the protruding olfactory apparatus on your face, or consider it to be your proudest feature, this device shapes your memory, learning, life and relationships like nothing else.

The nose is often relegated to the ignobility of being a resting place for eyeglasses or a conduit for ingesting illicit substance and medication. Despite such a lack of respect, it has a great deal of responsibility from breathing, smelling and taste, speech and the production of nasal vowels and consonants. In conjunction with the eustachian tubes, the nose plays a vital role in the pressure equilibrium maintained around the eardrums. It also has a secret opening to siphon excess tears, via the nasolacrimal ducts, which is why you have a runny nose when you cry. Finally, if you're a child then the nose offers extra storage capacity. It's not designed for this purpose, of course. As a doctor, I've lost count of the number of times I've had to extract small objects from this dual-piped orifice.

As the gateway to the life-giving respiratory realm, there's a lot riding on the nose. When it's not propelling juice out of its hole when you sneeze, or keeping loved ones awake when you snore, it's helping you to take in oxygen to the tune of 9 litres of air per minute. At the same time, it purifies each intake of air by producing plenty of mucus to filter out harmful compounds and microscopic fiends. The nose is truly the unsung Amazon of your anatomy, and like that precious rainforest, we fail to register what a vital role it has to be play in our existence.

Shorter, sharper, sleeker, snazzier ...

As the defining physical feature of the face, the nose gets its sweet revenge for this lack of respect by callously manipulating the self-esteem, confidence and self-image of millions of people worldwide. This nasal fixation is music to the ears of plastic and ENT surgeons, who perform expensive rhinoplasties (nose jobs) for patients hoping it'll improve their quality of life.

It might surprise you to know that rhinoplasties aren't a new-fangled fad. The origins of the procedure can be traced back to India in the sixth century BC. There, Ayurvedic practitioner Sushruta performed a crude attempt at reconstructive surgery to help people who'd had their schnozzes hacked off as a form of punishment for criminal acts. His work was so ahead of its time that the procedure was parked for many centuries in favour of special masks that people could wear to hide what remained of their noses, which was especially pertinent in sixteenth-century Europe when syphilis defiled and rotted such appendages. It wasn't until the late nineteenth century that American otolaryngologist, John Roe, reintroduced the rhinoplasty as a cosmetic procedure to enhance the appearance of a perfectly normal nose.

Nose vs mouth

Although the nose, nostrils and nasal cavity are key structures to facilitate our adventures in breathing, there is another contender for this spot – the mouth. In the battle between the two face holes, however, there is only one clear winner for several reasons.

When not moonlighting as a breathing apparatus, the mouth has another occupation. It's primary function involves eating and drinking. When it takes on the additional role of breathing, chaos can ensue in the form of choking. In addition, the nose has the uncanny ability to humidify incoming air, serve as a filter and also add warmth before it reaches the lungs. The mouth has limited capacity on all such counts, and though you could arguably survive by breathing in this fashion, your lungs won't love it.

Perhaps the most important consideration comes down to the fact that nobody wants to be a mouth breather. Besides the social stigma, it triggers a cascade of consequences which can, over time, modify the shape of your face to your disadvantage. Primarily, it means the muscles of the cheeks have to work harder, which puts more pressure on the upper and lower jaws. Over time this can narrow the shape of the face and the dental arches. This means there's less room in the mouth for the tongue, which drops to the floor from its natural resting position at the roof. This can be a particular concern in children, because if the tongue is down at the floor of the mouth it then it hinders the mid-face development. It means some youngsters who are chronic mouth breathers can end up with longer, narrower faces and even breathing issues and infections.

Time sharing

Your nose and its adjunctive structures are the input and output channels to your lungs. So, yes they're unexpectedly important but what disappoints me is that the channels are one and the same. This means you are deprived of having a continuous supply of air. Instead, you're forced to surrender the nostrils as a time-sharing estate between the forces of inspiration and expiration. Would a one-way system like the digestive tract be more sensible to avoid the accumulation of dirt? Then again, it would be unwise to imagine the vulgarity that would ensue if the alimentary canal shared one route for input and output.

We also need to pay some attention to the placement and structure of your nose. One particular aspect, which on the surface seems like a sub-par design, is the fact that it protrudes from the face. This exposes the nose to all manner of dangers, from face plants to head butts. This is before we even register the fragile cartilaginous support system the nose uses to bridge it to the skull. If the nose is attacked, voluntarily by your fingers or by fast-flying foreign objects, it is susceptible to leaks in the form of bleeding. Thankfully, you can influence your anatomy to turn off the hosepipe, or at least reduce the flow.

When I was a kid, I never became friends with any children that I saw picking their nose or eating the gruesome contents. I didn't consider myself to be a monster, after all. My relationship with the nose grew even more particular during a family trip to Florence at the age of eleven. Without warning, on this hot day ,with an ice cream in hand, my nostrils started leaking. Upon looking down, I found it wasn't strawberry syrup on my scoop of vanilla but my own blood. I had sprung a leak, a nosebleed out of the blue, and the very fact that I remember this minor incident so clearly speaks volumes about how freaked out I can be by this appendage. (I appreciate you don't want to hear this from a surgeon, which is why I specialise in gut surgery.)

Save yourself

The simplest way to stem bleeding is to pinch your nose, sit up straight and then tilt your head slightly forward to stop the blood running down the back of your throat. This is in complete contrast to the oft-quoted urban myth that you should tilt your head back, which will do little to stem blood flow and could also risk choking as blood leaks into your gullet (blood is an excellent laxative so this may be accompanied by loose stool hours later). When you pinch the soft area at the front of your nose, known as Little's area, known as Kiesselbach's plexus, you put pressure on the arteries likely causing the bleed.

If you're still dripping despite applying this pressure, you could roll up a small piece of tissue and place it in the area between your gum and upper lip; this applies further pressure on the blood vessels supplying your nose. If all this fails, you can't go wrong with simple ice; when wrapped in cloth and placed against the bleeding nostrils, the blood vessels should vasoconstrict and narrow to stem the spurting.

Occasionally, if the nose is irritated or invaded by foreign objects even as seemingly harmless as pollen, your nose can go into superfluous panic mode. It then produces more than the usual amounts of mucus, leaving you with a 'runny nose' or equally perplexing 'stuffed nose' as though such a nasal lockdown with the intruder trapped inside will rectify the situation.

The nasal gardener

A stray finger up the nostril doesn't just risk causing damage to the lining. It can also catch precious nose hairs and yank them out. While you might experience some orgasmic satisfaction in uprooting one of these nasal weeds, the catch is that it could kill you.

The problem with being your own nose gardener is that you're likely to be unaware of the different varieties. The tiny ones are known as cilia, and move mucus to the back of the throat for you to swallow. Yum. The larger, braver ones that stick their head out are known as vibrissae. These serve as the gatekeepers to deter unwanted guests. Plucking out any hair at the root results in a small opening that can allow microbes to gain entry to your innards and potentially cause an infection. One such risk relates to the Triangle of Danger on your face. This is the area between the corners of your mouth and nose, where any infection can cause serious problems. This is because the same veins that carry blood from the nose coalesce with those that transport blood from the brain. If you're unlucky, germs can hitch this secret backchannel to cause inflammatory anarchy in and around the brain, such as meningitis or brain abscesses. So, never pop a pimple that resides in the danger triangle!

The good news is that infections that start from a stripped nose hair are rare. Even so, they do occur and can be particularly serious for those with weakened immune systems.

Down with decongestant

If you sometimes struggle with a stuffy nose, science has a few tricks for you. A nasal decongestant contains a chemical which is a vasoconstrictor. This narrows the blood vessels to reduce blood flow, which works in the opposite way to Viagra (which increases blood flow to erectile tissue). It might sound like a random comparison, but for some lovers the act of coitus triggers a stuffy nose, known as honeymoon rhinitis.

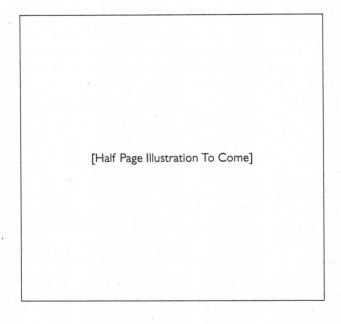

[Half Page Illustration To Come]

If you prefer not to use chemicals to clear a blocked nose, you could throw a towel over your head and gently breathe in steam from a bowl of hot (but not boiling) water, or use a nasal irrigation device, which is sometimes called a neti pot. One warning I will give with such irrigation tools would be to avoid using cold tap water to avoid the risk of pathogens entering your nose–brain blood circulation system. There have been instances of naegleria fowleri (a brain-eating amoeba) finding their way in through the nose, so decongest with respect.

Save yourself

The chemist's shelves might be crammed with decongestant products, but you could always opt for the far safer home alternative that is peppermint. The active ingredient is menthol, which actually acts as a natural nose unclogger.

Alternatively, you can always leverage your weird nose anatomy in order to breathe easier. Push your tongue to the roof of your mouth while pressing between your eyebrows for 20 seconds. Applying gentle pressure to both areas at the same time mobilises the vomer bone, which runs through the nasal passages. This motion loosens congestion and allows the sinuses to drain.

Why does a nose run?

Your nose is never satisfied. If blocked noses weren't enough of a nuisance, it likes to go to the opposite extreme by letting it run. We're talking about nasal diarrhoea, which is formerly known as rhinorrhea.

The salty torrents that wash down your upper lip via your face holes can be miserable, but it happens for a valiant reason. In the cold, without this extra moisture afforded by a runny nose, your nasal passages would dry out and become ripe for takeover by hostile microscopic predators and irritation. In some ways, the constant sniffing and sleeve-wiping is a small price to pay.

A runny nose can also happen when pathogens have snuck past the mucus lining. In response, in a bid to protect the body, your immune system stirs into action. It releases cytokines, which instruct cells in the nose to create more mucus to rid it of harmful microcritters. As a result, the snot factory goes into production overdrive, filling your nasal cavity with excess fluid that subsequently seeks a run-off.

Making sense of mucus

For all the negative press that mucus gets, it really is a multi-purpose body juice. It doesn't just serve as a first line of defence against an army of foreign invaders; among its many roles, far from the nose (I hope), mucus serves to keep sperm clumped together and allows smooth movement of poo by reducing friction. Quite simply, snot is the lubricant of life. When you're sick, the mucus production line speeds up so invaders can be trapped in suspended animation, which really means you should go easy on your nose when it clogs or runs away with you.

You can discern a lot by inspecting your nasal snot. For those inclined to admire your own produce, you aren't a freak. You are simply monitoring your health. Typically, mucus from the nose is clear. A yellow tinge is an indication of a smouldering infection your body is fighting, while green offers a suggestion of a bacterial infection that is momentarily winning the tug of war with your health.

Mucus is your ally, and yet it can sometimes be hijacked by the very creatures your body seeks to destroy. In their lust for spreading, viruses can travel in mucus and spread when you sneeze without covering your nose or push around a shopping trolley by a handle previously pawed by some grotty, snotty child. Whether it's serving to protect or kill you, mucus is a fact of life and good hygiene is the surest means to steer the odds in favour of your survival.

Nasal relay

Blocked noses don't just occur when you're sick or if nasal linings are inflamed. They are partially blocked all the time, and yet it doesn't feel like an issue until you're sick. Most of the day, you naturally breathe more heavily from one dominant nostril. Every couple of hours, one nostril takes over from the other with the heavy lifting. This system is known as the nasal cycle.

In order to alternate, your body inflates the lining of one nostril – which contains the same erectile tissue as found in the nether regions – with blood. This engorged erectile tissue subsequently causes congestion in one nostril for a few hours before switching sides. Why does the body do this? Well, the engorgement process helps to retain water and humidify the air you breathe. It also protects the delicate inner lining of your nasal cavities. It's an effective system to maintain both nasal health and inhaled air quality, and yet it's only when you're unwell or have allergies and one nostril is blocked that the switching cycle becomes both apparent and problematic.

Overflow drain

To keep your system of facial ventilation under some control you have a set of secret pipes in your skull. The sinuses are frequently no friend to humans. The mere description of them sparks ridicule. Cavities in your head which are filled with pathogen-trapping snot? Is that the best that Mother Nature could do? Even though sinuses clearly do some work, you only become aware of their fiendish existence when they erupt into dysfunction. Which they do frequently. Sometimes, sinuses make your life so miserable that you need surgery to restrain them . . . which involves drilling holes in your skull.

To illustrate the idiocy of such structures, when you stand upright the maxillary sinus behind your cheeks drains upwards. I mean who would design a system with liquid exit pipes at the top, thus resisting the universal force of gravity itself? You might think this can be rectified by tipping yourself forward like a teapot and emptying your sinus of mucus, but of course this is where your cavernous system of sinuses gets complex; once it drains out of one sinus it enters another – for example the ethmoid and frontal sinuses. So, no matter how you orientate yourself, you will always fill up another sinus with snot. My advice is that the next time you have a cold, don't feel sorry for yourself. Get angry. It's fine to be annoyed when you feel the mucus clawing into every facial orifice. Your maxillary sinus is heavily constipated, with a drainage hole hoping to work by defying gravity. Seriously, this isn't going to win any awards.

For the sake of balance, I can give your sinuses some credit. The goal is never to completely empty them completely. This is because their main role is to supply the nasal cavity with a steady supply of antibiotic-infused mucus to protect the body against microbes, dust and pollutants from the air. I still think the system could be refined, but then perhaps it is a demonstrably good thing the drain holes are at the top instead of the bottom. Otherwise, all the mucus would end up in your oral cavity because the base of the maxillary sinus sits just behind and below the nose, on top of the hard palate above the mouth. Potentially, it would create a socially awkward and perma-messy situation.

Thankfully, to fight the effects of gravity, your body has a hidden, ingenious and hard-working troop of labourers known as microcilia. These are little hairs that move mucus around to the appropriate drainage channels. So, the hole in the upper wall of the sinus serves as an overflow, just like you have in baths and sinks, which prevents catastrophic floods. In fact, if the holes of the sinus walls were placed at the bottom, it wouldn't just lead to excessively fast emptying. It would also cause the inner lining of the sinuses to dry out and become prone to blocking by mucus debris. In this view, you could even say that the upper overflow port is a sign of smart, higher thinking.

As a structure, the nose and its associated pipes are bewildering. What might look like flaws always seem to exist for a reason, and contributes to this being one of your oddest body parts. There are just so many components to the nasal system that serve several seemingly mismatched functions. So, while the sinuses might be an excellent conduit for snot, they also help the nose in an ability that's both essential and yet sometimes enough to make us gag. And that's your sense of smell.

The sniff test

You can walk into a stranger's house and immediately know whether someone is baking a cake, grilling some meat on a barbecue or had just dropped a fart wrongly thinking they were all alone. Smelling is more than just a side effect of breathing. It is as detailed as allowing you to smell the earthy scent of soil after heavy rainfall, known as petrichor, as well as the aroma of freshly cut grass on a summer's day. Pure witchcraft.

Anatomists, philosophers of yesteryear and early scientists were less than enthusiastic about your spectacle-holding mid-facial protuberance. Smell often had connotations of something bestial: pigs shoving their noses into the ground hunting for truffles or bloodhounds ferociously tracing scents in contrast to superior, upright, bipedal humans with their noses – literally – high above the ground. This disdain for the nose and sense of smell was discounted to such a degree that even Paul Broca, the nineteenth-century neuroscientist, was convinced the reason your olfactory bulb (smell neurons) were so small was because your brain didn't rely on smell. In this light, notable scientists relegated your sense of smell and its parental organ, the nose, to the ranks of vestigial appendages; a somewhat handy but ultimately useless piece of equipment.

The unseen smell

Our sense of vision and hearing rely on receptors that read light and sound waves respectively. These aren't tangible things. You can't touch sight or sound, which is where your sense of smell comes into its own.

Essentially, there is a chemical element behind every aroma, which is what our smell receptors can detect. Some noses aren't just attuned to pick up on the scent of roses or kebabs. Many creatures produce smells (beyond farts) as an important if poorly understood modulator of how they feel (for example, fear or arousal), the state of their hormones and even their health in general. These are called pheromones. Whether or not pheromones exist in humans is controversial. What is undeniable, however, is that you secrete various chemicals in tears, sweat and even breath that can influence the biology of others, and I'm not just talking about your pungent demonic morning breath forged in the ninth circle of hell. Mostly, it's a subtle process, beyond your control, but sometimes it's nice to think you're giving off fragrant vibes that can subconsciously strike the right notes with other people. A pipe dream. Perhaps.

How do you smell?

Humans have tried everything possible to defeat smell and create a deodorised society. We have become animals that don't want to smell like one, and wage war on bad breath, body odour, cheesy feet smell and sweat. Before the advent of the microscope, we even blamed disease and pestilence on nasty niffs and unpleasant aromas – also known as miasmas. In fact, we have an entire lexicon dedicated to a derided smell: stench, whiff, stink, pong, reek, funk, malodour, fetor, niff, hum, guff and so on.

Smells and scents are entrenched to your neurology tighter than a co-dependent couple and provide us with life-saving biases. Bad smells typically hint at some danger. So, they take a shortcut via the brain's fear processing centre – the amygdala – an emotional, direct, fear-infused control room, primal and animalistic. Good or neutral smells are associated with higher thinking power and nuance. These are processed in the cortex, the brain's outer layer, where they can be appreciated.

Take a sniff of the room you're in, but don't make it too obvious. Easy right? In reality, smelling is a surprisingly complex neurological process. You have smell-specific olfactory neurons in the nasal cavity that detect particles in the air from objects. These convey information via long nerve fibres through the skull into the brain that processes and makes sense of it. What is incredibly mind-boggling is that this adaptable system completely regenerates every six weeks, shedding the old olfactory neurons, creating brand new ones from scratch, and then reconnecting them with the brain tissue. Sometimes, however, this process can go wrong, temporarily or permanently, resulting in an inability to smell called anosmia.

Led by the nose

Despite the complexities, your sense of smell remains somewhat limited compared to other creatures. Although you can occasionally smell something at a great distance, it offers very limited navigational value and is all too easily scuppered by allergies, colds and infections that shut your sniffer down. Compared to the big boys of sound and vision, it's fair to say that smell is one of the lowest ranked senses. It's the kid that got picked last in school playground games, and the one people forget about. It was only during the Covid pandemic, when people suffered the curious condition of anosmia, that we came to realise that a world without smell is just not the same. We're talking about a sense that can influence your state of mind and affect your decisions. Just think of those sneaky estate agents filling rooms and houses with the scent of freshly baked cookies to lure you into parting with your cash. Potentially, that's an expensive mistake.

Too much of a good thing?

You have a nose that can detect a wide variety of smells, and yet it's surprisingly easy to deceive. For example, human waste includes some fascinatingly fragrant compounds like skatole. Skatole plays a large part in making poo smell, even though in low concentrations the same floral notes can be found in flowers like roses. It is even used in perfumes, and you made indeed regret reading this sentence should you like to dab a little eau de toilette behind the ears.

Indole is another compound found in poo. It also invokes the smell of death, decomposition and sex – a carnal, primordial crotch-like smell. So, naturally perfumers often add it to their products. Like skatole, the key to making sure the smell doesn't make your eyes water – but instead conjures an air of mystique and sophistication – is in the concentration. The fact is that in very small doses these compounds are interpreted in the brain as somewhat desirable. How can nature torture your confused nose in such a way? The answer remains a scientific mystery. It may be that when these chemicals enter your nose in large concentrations they bind to a wide range of smell receptors and overwhelm them. It isn't just high concentrations of poo compounds that trigger this response. Often, any intense smell can seem like too much, which simply reinforces the fact that your delicate nose is quite a special flower.

Save yourself

You can lose your sense of smell for all manner of reasons. More often than not, it's a temporary measure caused by a viral infection like Covid. Common colds can also cause the mucus membranes in the nostril to become irritated or blocked, as can some medication and antihistamines. Losing your sense of smell can sometimes be an underlying marker for high blood pressure or some illnesses, so it's always worth checking out with your GP.

Just like going to the gym to improve your strength, you can give your beak a workout. This can pay dividends if you've lost your sense of smell and are in need of rehab. Just be warned, it isn't fun. It's tedious, in fact, but the price to pay if you want smell back in your life.

On a basic level it involves sniffing potent aromas and scents several times a day. You might need to persist with this over weeks and even months to rewire, retrain and potentially even restore your damaged olfactory system.

Begin with a few powerful scents that evoke a specific mood or memories. It could be a favourite perfume, a shampoo or the aroma of coffee beans. Smelling each scent for up to 30 seconds with short, sharp sniffs rather than deep inhales is key, while also focusing on a mental image of when you last encountered it. The aim is to help reconnect or strengthen lines of communication between your brain and the olfactory

---

system. Effectively, smell training helps to trigger and potentially enhance the turnover of specialised nerve cells that can restore your sniffer.

Smells and memories

The key sensing structure within your nose is the olfactory bulb. Located a couple of centimetres above the roof of your mouth, it's a collection of neurons that are extensions from your brain into the mucosal lining on your nose. Physically, the neurons have 'hairs' or little feelers known as dendritic extensions that process smell within the mucus swamp of the mucosal lining and react to different odours.

The strangely wonderful thing (although sometimes not so great) is the association between smell and memory. These olfactory neurons delve into the brain like weeds and actually split off into different paths. One path contributes to an innate odour response, and this is hard-wired for survival purposes. Perhaps it helped our predecessors remember the location of a food source or danger area. One example would be neurons that respond to the smell of smoke. This is an adaptive function to help us detect something burning, because obviously that implies danger.

Some smells will be associated with appetite and hunger. In most cases, and particularly if you're hungry, the aroma of a freshly baked cake will evoke desire and prompt you to drop what you're doing in search of a slice. Once again, it's an innate pathway that requires no learning but is encoded in your software to help you survive in some way.

Save yourself

The simple act of smelling can actually improve cognitive function and thus enhance your memory and learning if used appropriately. It all comes down to inhaling and nose breathing rather than mouth breathing, which has implications for your brain as much as it does for your facial and jaw structure.

In contrast to breathing out, every time you inhale the upswing in your heart rate increases alertness and attention. Additionally, in breathing in we waft chemicals into our receptors to detect our environment. So, the act of inhaling becomes a cue to trigger the rest of the body to stand to attention. In short, the brain wakes up. There aren't any specific protocols for inhaling, but perhaps by varying the intensity and duration of your breath intakes – for example, a short burst of shorter, sharper intakes – might provide some modest enhancement during periods of learning or focus.

Beyond smell

Chances are you're blissfully unaware that you have four nostrils instead of two. I guess nobody (except me) has told you about the two internal ones at the back of the nasal cavity by the throat. Once you're over feeling like a freak, the good news is that you can use these secret nasal pipes to your advantage to boost your sense of taste. Yes, taste. Because the fact is that taste isn't really down to your tongue. Even without it, you'd still be able to taste most of what you eat, and that's because your sense of smell accounts for 80 per cent of the perception of flavour.

As you chew food, some of the airborne molecules wafting around your mouth pass through what is basically the back door of the nose. From there, your brain processes the odours of what you're eating. You can boost your taste by holding your food in your mouth for a bit longer and breathe out through your nose so the aromas percolate through these internal nostrils for longer. Indeed, we might yet make a sommelier out of you.

[Half Page Illustration To Come]

Health Hack

Closing the toilet lid before you flush isn't just kind to your nostrils. Scientists have discovered that it can also keep your bathroom from becoming engulfed in a mist of microscopic poo particles.

On flushing with the lid open, the sudden influx of water into the bowl causes a geyser of tiny droplets to rise up at a speed of 2 metres per second before fanning wide in a faecal mushroom cloud. Needless to say, this is probably sufficient information for you to cap your toilet after every visit as if your life depended on it.

9. Chewing on Nettles

A TRIP THROUGH TASTE

FROM THE OVERLOOKED POWER OF THE NOSE, we move to the unfairly exalted sense of taste. Yes, it enriches our lives, but taste uses the crutch of smell, visual input from the eyes and is sometimes even influenced by sounds to function. It pretends to be a cultured food critic while secretly checking what everyone else has to say.

Taste has done a great job in making out it's an invaluable sense, but does little to protect you in the same way as sight, smell and sound. We know to run away from a lion if we hear or see one. When it comes to poisons, which present a different kind of threat, taste demands that we put it in our mouth to detect if it's going to kill us. As a tool for survival, there is a flaw here that really should come with a warning sticker. Everything is edible, but some things only once.

Taste zones

When I expanded my knowledge of medicine, as a student and then a doctor, I realised a significant proportion of what I was taught in biology at school was incomplete at best. At worst, it was a damn lie.

One of the apocryphal myths I was seduced into believing claimed that the tongue has different taste zones. I vividly remember that my old biology textbook contained a diagram of an illustrated tongue marked out into different compartments: sweet at the front, bitter at the back, sour at the rear edges and salty on the sides towards the tip. This myth was further reinforced by a simplistic experiment in which we placed foods rich in these different flavours on those specific tongue zones. It didn't confirm the accuracy of the map for me, however, and I failed that lesson.

Thankfully modern science has come to my rescue by providing convincing evidence that the tongue boasts around 8,000 taste buds, all of which contain receptors that allow them to detect sweet, sour, salty and bitter and even the recently discovered umami, which is often described as savoury. Revenge is sweet.

While its talent in discerning flavours is undeniable, it seems your taste buds can perform too much of a good job. We all know vegetables are good for you but why didn't the design ensure they tasted as nice as all the sugars, fats and salts we actually love to gorge on? Now eat your greens.

Can we get a drink in here?

Without being synched with your other senses, your tongue receptors are somewhat compromised. As a stand-alone device, the tongue can be fussy and particular. First of all, the chemoreceptors in your taste buds require the chemicals in the food you are eating to be dissolved in order to bind to the receptors. This means a liquid medium is necessary. Before you reach for the beer, I'm talking about saliva.

Your taste buds are certainly responsible for your perception of taste, but without saliva to break down the molecules that make up the chewing gum you've just shoved into your mouth it won't be detected. You can try this for yourself. Dry your tongue with a paper towel and then pop something tasty on to your tongue. Until your salivary glands lubricate the oral lab, that sample will be devoid of taste. What's key here are the enzymes swimming in your saliva that deconstruct the food and release molecules, which are finally analysed by your taste buds.

In a reversal of flavour fortune, a particular enzyme in pineapple called bromelain actually breaks down the protein on your tongue, lips and inner lining of your cheek. This is why you get that fuzzy sensation when you eat it because you're literally being digested by pineapple.

Illusions of the tongue

Your tongue is led astray by many fallacies, illusions and acts of deceit. If you've ever guzzled some orange juice after brushing your teeth with toothpaste then it's likely that you've also been ambushed by a strange flavour. Your tongue is tricked by an ever-shifting oral environment; foods you ate previously leave their stains on the canvas of your tongue – for better or worse – and that impacts on the flavour of what you eat next.

To understand why your tongue is so gullible, it's worth understanding what exactly happens once a food molecule presents itself to a taste receptor. These are tiny, highly sensitive cells that contain proteins on their surface that act like doorbells. So, when a specific food molecules presses the buzzer, it rings in the brain to provide one of the big five taste sensations.

It's a simple procedure, and yet the limitation of your tongue means it isn't also fail-safe. Take the artichoke, for example, which has the ability to run rings around your flapping mouth appendage. Within this clever vegetable resides the chemical cynarine, which fixes itself to the sweet receptors when you eat some but doesn't stimulate them. As soon as you swig some water, however, the cynarine molecules are washed away, thus releasing these receptors. Freed to function at last, the receptors send a message to the brain to generate a sweet taste, and yet by then chances are the mouthful of artichoke is snaking down your oesophegus on its digestive journey. So, in effect, you're left with a taste that's late to the mouth party.

The failure of the tongue to stand confidently on its own doesn't end there. We know your brain, the sneaky producer behind the scenes, integrates various data from the main five senses to produce a partially coherent version of reality. Often, there is significant overlap between how these senses can influence each other as they bubble up to your consciousness stream. You've salivated at the sight and smell of your favourite food, but perhaps less well known is the influence that sound can have on taste.

Save yourself

Your tongue isn't just about taste. In many cases, it's also a screen of your inner health. Just like other parts of your body, your tongue can be affected by systemic illness manifesting in physical changes. This floppy meat stick in your mouth won't help you diagnose everything but it can be a telling early warning sign for illness, disease and infection.

Open your mouth, stick out your tongue and peek in the mirror.

- A normal, healthy tongue is typically pink and covered in small bumps called papillae.

- A black, hairy tongue – while shocking to see – could indicate poor oral hygiene, diabetes or be as a result of cancer treatment. Occasionally, it can be caused by an accumulation of dead skin cells, which can be removed by gently brushing with a toothbrush.

- A strawberry-coloured tongue that is larger than usual could suggest a B12 iron or folate deficiency. In some children it could be a sign of a streptococcal infection.

- A tongue that is coated in white patches is usually a tell-tale sign of oral candidiasis, a yeast infection, which can be effectively treated by checking in with your GP.

The Pringle experiment

To confirm his suspicions regarding the influence of sound on taste, Charles Spence, a professor of experimental psychology at Oxford

University, conducted a strange experiment using the more-ish, addictive, paraboloid snack known as the Pringle.

In turn, Spence invited twenty participants to don a pair of headphones and take their places in front of a microphone in a soundproof booth. Then, each participant was instructed to bite into 200 Pringle crisps (chips if you're American, or cake if we're to believe the judge who ruled on the 2008 British court case seeking to define the product). With every single crunch, the test subjects gave a crispiness and freshness rating according to what they could hear from the sound looped from the microphone into their headphones.

Unbeknown to the participants, Spence mutated the native crunching noises. He did so by using an amplifier and equaliser to either dampen or boost various frequencies to alter the sound. At the end of this bizarre experiment, the subjects were asked if all the cak . . . crisps were the same.

Despite being identical Pringles, the subjects reported subjective differences; some were less fresh, some were crisper. Upon analysis, Spence correlated that the Pringle crunch sounds associated with a louder, higher-pitched noise led participants to perceive a freshness increase of 15 per cent over the unamplified crisps. This was the first (documented) experiment of its kind to demonstrate that sound alone could alter taste. In an elegant way, this seemingly weird test showed the strange way two sensory inputs – the tactile oral feel of a Pringle and a distinct crunching sound – could be manipulated into one multisensory perception, which to some degree is something all your senses are involved in.

It is tempting to view each sense as possessing one role. In fact, the vast majority of research into the subject has focused on how each sense functions independently. It's a theory that seems to fit until we reach taste, which can work alone but just isn't very good. Taste only comes into its own, in fact, when it calls upon multisensory inputs for back-up.

So, what you perceive as flavour is merely a tangible illusion of the tongue. In many ways it's a filtered olfactory process with the taste buds playing second fiddle. We could go further to state that the majority of your gastronomical experiences are determined by the forgotten flavour organs of the eyes, ears, brain and tactile sensations.

Charles Spence did not stop with his Pringles experiment. He's conducted many world-changing tests, proving – among other things – that strawberry mousse tastes sweeter when eaten from a white container versus a black one; that coffee taste less sweet when drunk from a white mug as opposed to a clear one; and that soup served from blue containers makes it seem significantly saltier.

Spence's experiments have even inspired an entire field of gastronomical cooking. In 2006, celebrity chef Heston Blumenthal co-conducted an experiment with him to demonstrate the flavour of bacon was more 'bacony' when accompanied by the acoustics of sizzling bacon. In fact, Blumenthal created a 'sound of the sea dish' at his Michelin-starred restaurant, The Fat Duck, that was served with beachside sounds to boost the flavour of the meal. Perhaps all roads will eventually lead to the use of sound to help improve the lives of the elderly, as your sense of taste diminishes with age.

Trust nothing

The illusory nature of taste is perfectly epitomised by *Synsepalum dulcificum*, a plant that produces a small red fruit dubbed the miracle berry.

This unassuming fruit has a pleasantly tangy taste, but the real fun begins when you follow it up by biting into a lemon or lime. Then, rather than causing your entire face to pucker, your mouth is flooded by a paradoxical sensation of sweetness. This is because your taste buds are deceived by miraculin. It's the active compound in the berry that binds to the sweet receptors and blocks them. Then, when your saliva becomes acidic thanks to the citrus fruit, the miraculin changes its structure and triggers the same sweet receptors it was previously blocking.

The very same taste illusion is similarly replicated by the body when you have sinus issues and nasal problems. They can distort your sense of taste to leave you perceiving normal food items like coffee or vanilla as putrefaction, death and decay. This is dysgeusia. Disgusting.

Benign masochism

In talking about taste we must bring spice to the table. We're talking the hot stuff here, like chillies and the kind of sauce that only 'real men' can handle on their hot dogs. At least that is the macho cultural myth that surrounds this much misunderstood foodstuff.

To begin, let me just state that if you love spicy food then you might be just a tiny bit kinky. Let me explain your dark secret . . .

'Spicy' is not a taste. Your tongue can only determine sweet, salty, bitter, sour and umami when it comes to informing the brain of what's in your mouth. At the same time, however, your tongue can also determine pain and temperature, which is how spicy food makes its presence known. This is down to the chemical capsaicin, an active component of chilli peppers, which binds to taste receptors and ignites that hot sensation.

You could say it's a weird form of benign masochism, in that you like pain but not too much of it. In fact, if you eat a lot of spicy food this has the effect of desensitising pain receptors. As a result, you find yourself seeking spicier food in a doomed bid to feel the burn, which is why capsaicin is sometimes used to treat chronic pain.

When you eat spicy food, your tongue is tricked into thinking your mouth has spontaneously ignited. Your body is unaware that it's not a real threat, and so it responds by sweating in an attempt to cool off. At the same time, a series of physiological changes occur to release vasodilatory substances to widen your blood vessels. Your body is equipped with TRPV1 receptors, which can bind to capsaicin, including in the area around your anus. So, any capsaicin molecules that find their merry way down your GI tract will eventually cause the dreaded ring sting. You have been warned.

Save yourself

Water won't help you banish the chilli demons. If the heat becomes too much and you need to extinguish the fire in your mouth, water could actually make things worse.

Water consists of what are called polar molecules, with positive and negative ends, while capsaicin has a non-polar structure. This means when you mix capsaicin and water, the chemical is not broken down. It requires another non-polar substance to do that, such as milk and other dairy products.

If you're looking for a simple way to reduce your snacking, minimise snacking when you have a blocked nose. Our sense of smell is crucial to our brains' overall ability to achieve a feeling of satisfaction and fullness, so people with blocked noses tend to consume more food than necessary because it's not satisfying enough.

For those who usually add sugar to their tea or coffee, you might want to use a red-coloured mug. Our brains are wired to associate colours with flavours: green for bitter, yellow for sour, brown for savoury and red for sweet. A red mug will allow you to add less sugar and still feel that it's sweet enough. Likewise, adding vanilla to desserts allows bakers to use less sugar because we associate the aroma of vanilla with sweetness.

To reduce sugar in your coffee, you could add salt. What happens next is an illusion – salt doesn't actually do anything to the coffee itself but it tricks your brain into ignoring the bitterness. You have thousands of taste buds in your tongue responsible for recognising the five basic tastes: sweet, salt, bitter, sour and umami. Salt can amplify all of them except bitterness. When you taste bitterness, your taste buds release calcium ions. Salt actually overrides this biology to help mask bitterness in the coffee and at the same time amplifies the sweetness. This works really effectively in things like salted caramel. If you're sensitive to bitterness or find black coffee too bitter you can actually add salt to the coffee grounds itself or even the brew.

[Half Page Illustration To Come]

Health Hack

Ripe and unripe bananas have different health benefits. Here's how to hack the best from your favourite fruit:

* The greener, younger variety contain a higher proportion of resistant starch. This is a form of carbohydrate that acts like a fibre. It's a prebiotic that your gut loves to consume.

* What's more, the greener your banana the lower its glycaemic index. This means it takes longer for your body to break it down into glucose, so you'll get a slower, more gradual release of energy.

* A yellow, riper banana is easier to digest. This is because over time more starch is converted into simple carbohydrates.

* A brown, or overripe, banana might not seem as appealing to some, but it contains a higher antioxidant content due to a breakdown in the chlorophyll pigment.

10. What a Feeling

HOW TOUCH CAN
TAKE YOU OUT

YOUR SENSE OF SIGHT, hearing, smell and taste all share the same basic blueprint. They occupy a small, concentrated area of your body, which contains a collection of densely packed receptors. They are as sophisticated and as slung together as each other, and yet all of them have to bow down to a beast of a sense that outshines them all, and that sense is touch.

Like a parasite, touch receptors have invaded all parts of your body from your fingertips to your nether regions. Depending on the area, and the way in which these receptors are activated, touch can produce a dazzling array of emotions. It is quite different from the other senses and perhaps this is where it fails you. How? Well, it is overly reliant on mechanical pressure and can't detect incoming signals like light, sound or even chemicals until it's too late. It is, however, far better than the rest of the senses at investigating your own body rather than your external environment.

Can't touch this

It's arguably your most important sense, on the front line of how you interact with the physical world, and yet touch is just an illusion. I'm not trying to be mystical or philosophical here. It's a fact. The explanation comes down to physics. Electrons exist in every atom, and so when you 'touch' something, the electrons in your fingertips effectively repel those in the item you're touching. The sense of touch you feel is in fact your brain registering a disruption in the electromagnetic field. So, it turns out you aren't sitting in that chair after all, but levitating at a microscopic level.

SKIN IN THE GAME

Your sense of touch is primarily overseen by one of the brutes of your body. The skin is the largest organ by surface area, and it literally envelopes you from head to toe. We're talking about your body's first line of defence against the outside world, a border guard — but one that often doesn't always do its job properly.

The skin is also somewhat maligned. You only have to think about the rigours of a skincare routine to think of it as kind of high maintenance, but it does also work hard for you. Without your skin, a sort of biological giftwrapping, you would lose precious water from your body and succumb to death and the deadly laser in the sky known as the sun would begin frying your deeper layers. Your skin, or the outermost cells which stoically guard you, expose themselves to harmful radiation to protect you. It's a self-sacrificial role to protect the other cells behind them.

Human armour

In number-crunching terms, your skin weighs around 10kg and typically consists of 15 per cent of your total body weight. The outer layer, known as the epidermis, is effectively a thin barrier that we take for granted, scratching, grazing, pinching, pulling and stretching it thousands of time a day without it wearing out. This is because your skin is alive (sort of). The cells on your skin surface are being constantly replenished with new building blocks known as keratinocytes. These are literally tough as nails. Indeed, the same substance can be found in the horns and claws of animals.

Keratinocytes are formed from stem cells that live in the bottom most layers of your epidermis. They rise up through the ranks and form a waterproof layer on reaching the surface to secure your skin from intruders and the environment. Eventually they draw their last breath and flake off into the air. However, if you stress out your skin too much, for example by excessive rubbing or abrasive forces, the epidermis goes over the top to produce new skin, resulting is unsightly calluses.

Unfortunately for you, your skin is more than just giftwrapping for your internal organs. The deeper layer underneath, the dermis, houses a large network of blood vessels, which is why you can bleed generously from superficial skin cuts. It also contains a large army of immune cells. They wait patiently to attack any foreign intruders, and are responsible for inflammation should you suffer an injury to the surface.

The surprises of the skin don't end there. One of the reasons you have elastic, stretchy skin that springs back is due to important proteins known as collagen and elastin. These same proteins which give your skin shape and plumpness also have the potential to betray you. If you're a smoker, or suffer from poor sleep or stress, these proteins can degrade to leave you wrinkly, etched with fine lines and bags under your eyes.

As a final point – and let's hope this isn't bedtime reading – you are not alone in your skin. It is in fact a microbiome crawling with billions of bugs, home to over a thousand varieties of bacteria. Some confer benefits to skin health, while others are nefarious and contribute to disease. Lights out?

Skinned alive

Just like the gut microbiome, research suggests that skin-directed probiotic treatments could help positively influence the health of the skin and tackle conditions like acne, psoriasis and eczema. Don't worry, faecal transplants for skin health won't be available any time soon (or ever, hopefully). Even so, the idea behind microbiota transplant – effectively rehousing bacterial populations from one person to another – might be an avenue to watch carefully. One case study of twins from 2017, one with bad BO and the other with none, showed how armpit microbes taken from the one who didn't smell could be transplanted as a means of 'curing' the other. Phew!

In similar fashion to your gut microbiome, these bugs are the middlemen between your immune system and the natural world. They help to modulate your immune system to reduce its overreaction to harmless threats and improve its efficiency at dealing with viable aggressors. Just as microbial biodiversity is much vaunted for your gut, such diversity is something to be sought for your skin. A wide range of exposure helps train your immune system through its interface with the microbes.

As much as I'd like to bad mouth the skin, the simple truth is that you aren't giving it due respect. The skin is your first battalion of defence against disease and yet you often stop the various organisms and bacteria on its surface from doing their important work by overzealously washing them away. Ultimately, the majority of the creatures renting real estate on your skin are harmless freeloaders that scavenge on your sweat, oil and dead skin cells without disrupting your daily routine. Furiously washing yourself just leads to the removal of the natural oils which lubricate your skin (sebum) and it's that which feeds the microbes. This resultant 'dysbiosis' of the skin microbiome might certainly have a role to play in the cause of allergic skin conditions like eczema.

One of the benign demons lurking on your skin is demodex. They're only a half millimetre in length but can stretch much, much further. Despite looking a bit like lice, they are in fact a type of arachnid that is colourless, has only four legs and burrows into the skin of your face and eyelashes. As horrific as this sounds, these nightmare bugs actually act as natural exfoliants as they feast on your sebum and dead skin cells. It's only if you host too many that they can cause skin disease and sleepless nights.

I probably shouldn't mention that these tiny face mites that call your skin home also have no anuses. As a result, they die from overconsumption from all the backed up skin and oil they've consumed. They also have sex on your face at night, like you're some kind of dogging site for mites.

Eventually these worm-spider looking creatures become increasingly bloated after gorging on your face and enjoying special time together. Then they explode and die.

About body odour

You might recoil at the pungent aroma of someone's body odour (BO) and perhaps occasionally be surprised by your own brand of stench. Despite possessing seemingly lethal properties, it is actually a by-product of a protective feature in your skin. This is courtesy of a bacteria known as bacillus subtilis – subtle in name only. On the ground (aka the skin) this bacteria produces antifungal chemicals by excretion, having ingested waste from your skin such as sweat and oils.

Then we come to your feet, unfortunately. Here, brevibacteria cause foot odour by ingesting dead skin cells and then producing a gas that produces a distinct sour, cheesy smell. This might leave a nasty taste in your mouth, and yet some cheesemakers add this bacteria to some cheeses to help develop the aroma and flavour. (Yes, I know.)

The balance of power

The skin is mostly an inhospitable wasteland. It's an expanse devoid of nutrients; dry and acidic. However, the lipid-dense hair follicles provide an oasis-like getaway in the desert of your skin. Despite these arid conditions, your skin microbiome strives to make do within this ecosystem. With resources scarce, some of the bugs that inhabit this neighbourhood engage in turf warfare. Take the bacteria staphylococcus epidermidis, which helps to protect against the malicious staphylococcus aureus. Depending on your lifestyle and environmental factors, you can disrupt the balance of power in an unfavourable way by making yourself more susceptible to skin break-outs or conditions like atopic dermatitis, a type of eczema. Even supposedly helpful bacteria species like cutibacterium acnes, which can typically produce chemicals that deter pathogens, have certain strains which have a causative role in the kind of acne nobody wants. Alliances are fickle. Trust no one.

We are still at a nascent stage of understanding the skin microbiome and what factors help determine whether a specific bacterial strain is a friend or foe. When we further our understanding, we may be able to forge new treatments where administration of skin bacteria from one person to another might help clear conditions like acne and atopic dermatitis.

Squeaky clean

The concept of hygiene and cleansing practices are as old as civilisation itself. In fact, the entire miasma theory of disease was largely based around the idea that poor hygiene was a result of contaminated water. While this obsolete theory was replaced by our understanding of germs, perhaps our obsession with hygiene and skincare rituals has gone too far in the opposite direction. While you may not want to hold out for weeks, months or years without cleansing yourself, the fact is your expensive and elaborate routines might cause more harm than help.

I won't lie to you. For a very long time I had no skincare routine. When I was twenty-one, I experimented with various creams and cleansers, not really having any idea what I was doing. Although I never suffered terribly with acne or blemishes, I gave up on the pursuit of glowing skin. In fact, throughout most of my twenties my skincare was limited to washing my face in the shower and applying sunscreen only if I went to the beach. Once I graduated from medical school, aware of the role the skin plays in keeping me alive and well, I decided it was worth making it more of a priority.

Save yourself

It's easy to feel overwhelmed by all the choices on offer when it comes to skincare, but it can be simplified. A good, healthy routine doesn't rely on gimmicks – It also doesn't need to cost a fortune, or take up hours of your time each day. In a nutshell, it comes down to washing your face regularly, moisturising and wearing a sunscreen every bloody day, which could eventually save your life. At the same time, it's worth noting that if you have specific concerns like severe acne, eczema or rosacea then check in with your GP. They may refer you to a dermatologist to help figure out what products benefit your condition, which will likely include prescription medication.

While we're here, let's also throw in some skin hygiene basics. I know you may find this idea horrific, but perhaps consider not taking your mobile phone into the bathroom with you when you go for your morning dump. Whether you like the visuals or not, your bathroom will be filled with microscopic faecal particles. They percolate the air and land wherever they please. It's more than likely these minute poo flakes will land on your phone screen, where they will quickly move from your swiping fingertips to your face as soon as you touch it. You can see where this is going.

It's worth pointing out that on average you touch your face upwards of twenty-three times an hour. While this is largely subconscious and inevitable, reducing the frequency of face touching will help reduce transmission of bacteria from the environment to your face. Your hands aren't messy infants, so instruct them to act their age.

What the doctor ordered

My bathroom shelf is relatively sparse. The main headline is that I use a cleanser. The active ingredients contained within cleansing products help to stick to oil on one end and water on the other and encase the oils in tiny bubbles called micelles, which can be washed away. Soap can do this job as well but the trouble is it can be too good and excessively strip away far too much of your skin's natural oils. I personally avoid those scrub-type cleansers that have tiny plastic beads or 'bits'. Not only can they be far too abrasive for most skins but they are also problematic for the environment.

Next on my shelf is a moisturiser. Maintaining or increasing the water content of your skin is unquestionably a good thing. Moisturising products work by keeping water in your skin so it looks and also probably feels plumper and fuller. But more importantly the skin will then be able to do a better job in acting as a barrier to the harms of your external environments. This is epitomised in skin conditions like eczema which flare up when skin is dry and settle when skin is well moisturised.

Arguably one of the design flaws of your skin is that every time you touch anything, you lose a few skin cells. However, this loss is mitigated by a continuous replacement of fresh cells that take their place. The top layer of skin that you see and touch with is called the stratum corneum. These are essentially dead skin cells joined together by bridges called desmosomes. The space between the cells is filled with lipids.

When your skin isn't moisturised, the enzymes which break the desmosome bridges, aren't as effective. This results in clumps of skin cells falling away rather than one skin cell at a time, which gives rise to the appearance of flaky skin. Moisturiser works to surround these enzymes with water to improve their effectiveness. It might also be useful to keep an eye out for a couple of specific ingredients in your moisturising product. Occlusives prevent water leaving the skin and humectants help draw water in from the deeper layers. A good moisturiser contains both.

I can't mention skincare without talking about sunscreen. Yes, you also need sunscreen when it's not sunny and if you have darker skin. It needs to be worn year round, every day, whether you plan to fry yourself on the beach or not. Aside from reducing the risk of skin cancer and preventing sunburns, sunscreen is one of the few genuine 'anti-ageing' products out there. It prevents thickening and wrinkles that occur with ageing skin. The sun protection factor (SPF) is a marker of how long the sunscreen can protect your skin from the UVB rays. The higher the rating the higher the percentage of UVB rays blocked. SPF 30 blocks around 97 per cent of UVB rays.

While my skincare routine goes back to basics – because I like to keep it real – what about those fancy products like masks and serums? The reality is that the purported benefits of most of these products are either completely shrouded in pseudoscience or foregrounded in a questionable bid to suggest how essential it is in improving your skin health. I don't want to stop you enjoying overly complicated routines and trying new products. Just as long as it doesn't harm your skin and you're aware that a simple routine is often the most effective.

Save yourself

In any skincare product, there are some common active ingredients which can help your skin. Keep your eyes peeled for the following:

- Salicylic acid helps exfoliate dead skin cells. It also works well on oily skin, which makes it a popular ingredient in anti-acne products.

- Alpha-hydroxy acids and benzoyl peroxide are also classic anti-acne agents that hit bacteria with free radicals.

- Retinoids are related chemically to vitamin A. They help to increase the turnover rate of skin and help you shed dead skin cells. Retinoid agents are effective against acne and are in their own right 'anti-ageing'.

[Half Page Illustration To Come]

Health Hack

It might seem a touch too far for some, but cleaning your bum hole with a cheeky finger whenever you shower or bathe could save you from a world of irritation and pain.

* As a gut surgeon, I examine rusty tailpipes on a daily basis. All too often – with the help of a glove and lubricant – a sweep of my finger encounters poo flakes that are the single biggest cause of pruritus ani, also known as 'itchy bum'.

* For most people, an itchy bum is an annoyance, but poor peri hygiene (as it's known) can lead to infections such as anal abscesses – basically an internal pimple that can hurt like hell.

11. Privates on Parade

THE INFERNAL GENIUS
OF GENITALS

TOUCH, PLEASURE, LUST, love and orgasms. While other creatures exist
to simply reproduce, it seems that humans are one of a handful of species,
alongside dolphins, bonobos and short-nosed fruit bats, that also engage
in the devil's dance for pleasure. We boast dangerously complex brains
capable of genius and incredible abstract thought, and yet it seems we use
this gift to engage in what is a bestial, primal act, above all because it's fun.
What's more, we do so with ample disregard for personal safety. In fact,
we barely give any thought to what we're doing at all.

It's worth noting that the desire to use your reproductive tools often
happens in tandem with a decreased brain function. In a sense, humans
become slaves to these natural pleasure orifices. For men and women, the
sex holes and bits and bobs that make up the body are remarkable in their
offerings, and yet they possess indelible limitations. These can be irksome,
and also prone to painful problems, which in some cases can be deadly.
So, consider this to be not so much a celebration of human genitalia but a
cautionary insight for men and women into how to prevent our privates
from killing us.

TACKLE TROUBLE AND
LETHAL WEAPONS

Sperm or snowflake?

One of the most conspicuous and hard-to-explain features of the male body is the fact that the testicles are external. Design-wise, they dangle precariously on the precipice of the pelvis: vulnerable, exposed, flapping in the wind.

Naturally there is an explanation. Human sperm cells require a strict range of temperature regulation for optimal activity and maturation; in some ways, the testicles are the biological equivalent of Goldilocks. They need an environment that isn't too hot or too cold, but just right. This precision demand is in the name of the sperm production going on inside, which is optimised some 3–4 degrees below the ideal body temperature of 98.6 degrees. An increase in scrotal temperature by even as little as 2 degrees can negatively affect sperm formation, reduce sperm count and the number of abnormal sperm. With this in mind, it makes complete sense to make them an exterior feature, in the same way that we might consider the patio to be an outside extension of the home.

To ensure they're not completely exposed to the elements, the testicles are suspended in an adjustable hammock. This is temperature-sensitive, which allows sperm cells to flourish just at the edge of the abdominal cavity; this human carrier bag is known as the scrotum. The muscles of the scrotum can expand and contract, adapting to temperatures and serving as a kind of quality regulator for the sperm production factory inside.

The testicles are an exception to the rule that human cells can live happily in the heated environment of the body. Blood cells grow inside bone marrow, ovaries are generated in the pelvis, so why then are sperm a law unto their own? They have a lot to answer for.

While the rest of the human organs stay tucked up safely inside, the testicles have a lot of nerve hanging outside like delinquents. Want to find the testicles on a frog? Well, you won't – unless you've got a scalpel handy because the sperm-creating kit for your cold-blooded relatives are safely tucked away on the inside. Meanwhile, a lot of mammals have the convertible testicle upgrade option enabled. Mice and rabbits can dangle their gonads so they're nice a cool on the outside when they want to breed, and then fold them in for safe keeping when surplus to requirements. This non-permanent fertility control would be handy for humans. Not only could it prevent the dire consequences associated with a kick to the groin, but it could also prevent unintended pregnancies and do away with the need for the apocryphal 'pull-out' method of contraception.

Perhaps we can argue that testicles are not just a chemical conduit for population growth but a mascot for it. It is not unreasonable to conclude that two conspicuous, well-advertised dangling tendrils of flesh provide some selective advantage when choosing mates.

A treacherous descent

Before they become susceptible to the forces of nature, the testicles begin life inside the body. As a young male foetus develops, and the body becomes too warm for its precious cargo, they embark upon a pilgrimage to the sunlit downlands of the nutsack. To begin, our pair of spherical wanderers set out from the abdomen somewhere near the kidneys. During gestation, they migrate downwards towards the pelvis while leaving an open tunnel behind them known as the inguinal canal. This descent causes problems, however. It leaves an open back channel through which structures from inside your abdomen – like sections of intestine or body fat – can protrude. These can result in groin (inguinal) hernias. It occurs far more frequently in men because women don't have their entire reproductive plumbing externalised. As a result, men are highly dependent on delicate pipework that passes from the inside to the outside of the body, which can invite unintended bits to follow suit. Thankfully, surgery has made hernias a largely treatable condition. Without intervention, they can cause chronic pain and even cut off blood supply to the intestines.

As the balls continue to drop, a tube known as the vas deferens can cause issues. It connects the testes to the urethra (pee pipe) and can becomes entangled with the ureter (a tube that carries urine to the bladder from the kidneys). At best, it's a haphazard structural arrangement. At worst, it's a knotty problem that could require urgent surgical attention.

Sometimes the testicular descent fails to happen altogether. This is known as cryptorchidism and surgically it's relatively straightforward to fix. Even so, children with cryptorchidism have a higher risk of testicular cancer in later life. This isn't believed to be caused by the fact that the testicles haven't dropped; rather, it's an indication of an abnormality in the testicle that is associated with cancer.

Save yourself

I was never taught how to play with my balls. That's a sentence I didn't think I'd write in published book but here we are. I'm not alone, however. Men are rarely taught how to properly examine their testicles to check for lumps, even though testicular cancer is one of the most curable types of cancers. It really is something worth doing on a weekly basis, if not more often.

The ideal time to check is during or after a hot shower. When it's cold, the dartos muscle in the scrotum contracts, making it hard to effectively feel the crown jewels, but during a hot shower, this muscle relaxes thus allowing you to have a better feel of the boys. Make sure you feel both at the top and the back of the testicle. You might feel a lump but it's likely to be the epididymis, which is the tube that transports sperm. There is no strict hard and fast rule but just know that one testicle usually hangs lower and is bigger than the other. If you do notice any swelling or lump that is growing in size or shape – even if painless – get it checked out.

Twist in the tale

Most horrifying hospital stories have their origins in a night shift. This one starts on my way home, as the first rays of sunshine competed with the last of the streetlights. As I dragged myself to my doorstep, the bat-phone (as the emergency on-call phone is known) started ringing. With a sigh (I was still on call), I picked up. From the other end of the line, the emergency room doctor frantically blurted out a monologue about a nine-year-old boy with a twisted testicle. Oh dear. I don't think nature ever intended nor expected the male balls to be inundated with the level of torturous pain yielded by testicular torsion. It's not an uncommon phenomenon, which generally occurs due to physical trauma to the crown jewels. Sometimes, however, it can happen through an odd movement or sheer bad luck. Whatever the cause, it can strangle the spermatic cord which carries the testicular blood supply. The result is not just unrelenting pain, but it also carries the high risk of losing a flesh marble. Left untreated, there is also a chance the unfortunate male will die.

When any tissue in the body is deprived of its oxygen supply for long enough, ischaemia follows. This is arguably the most painful biological process in the human body that mediates some of the most painful conditions humans can go through: labour, heart attacks, testicular torsion and even period pains. Ischaemia and poor tissue perfusion, if prolonged, can lead to tissue death known as necrosis. When testicular torsion is in play, the timer starts. You have approximately six hours to detort or untwist the testicles and restore the blood supply, otherwise one testicle will end up in the bin (after surgery of course).

I raced back to the hospital and reviewed the patient. The poor boy was in the paediatric department rolling around in agony. His left testicle seemed to be lying abnormally. I performed a test which involves stroking the inner thigh to elicit an involuntary response known as the cremasteric reflex. In a testicle functioning as it should, this causes a contraction in the cremaster muscle surrounding it. If this reflex is absent then it is invariably torsion we are dealing with. Having confirmed the pathology, I rushed the boy to the operating room; there, under general anaesthetic, my team and I fixed it by untwisting the testicle to restore blood flow and then suturing it to the interior wall of the scrotal sack to secure it in place. This is an operation known as an orchidopexy – orchi referring to testicle, pexy derived from the word to stitch. The procedure is fairly simple but time-critical, with (literally) a great deal hanging on it, as was evident in the sheer relief that lifted from the shoulders of his parents when I confirmed a happy outcome.

Save yourself

When it comes to optimising the temperature so sperm can thrive, men don't need to leave their testicles to do all the heavy lifting. As a man, if your job involves being in a warm or hot environment, and you're hoping to become a father, then consider taking regular breaks to cool off (including down below). Additionally, if you are sedentary (i.e. deskbound) for prolonged periods of time, then make sure you get up and move around frequently. Also steer clear of tight underwear, which is believed to raise testicular temperature slightly (in some cases by up to 1 degree).

Beyond temperature, protecting your equipment itself is crucial. You can do this by limiting the intake of various toxins that eventually percolate through to your sperm and affect their quality and number. These include recreational drugs such as cannabis, cocaine and alcohol. Stress is another culprit, which can not only lower libido (sex drive) but ultimately have an impact on testosterone.

On leaks and blockages

The urinary tract possesses some awkward and unusual wiring which, if you are a man, can make life a misery. The male urinary tract traverses directly through the prostate, a gland prone to enlargement with age or swelling due to cancer or infection. While unintentional, that makes prostate issues a prime cause of blockage when it comes to urine flow.

Inserting a collapsible tube through an apparatus that is highly prone to expanding and obstructing the flow of liquid through it is a terrible idea. In plumbing terms, it would never get signed off. If anyone discovers a reason why this arrangement exists, it will allow me to move the prostate to the bottom rung of organs that matter.

At some point, a significant proportion of men over the age of fifty will have prostate troubles. Some might end up requiring investigations, which can involve probing the urethra with metal objects and lasers, and even surgery. We've already taken the likes of the gall bladder and the pancreas to task for being downright dangerous at times. Compared to the prostate, however, these organs look saintly. This walnut-sized organ produces prostatic fluid, which sounds essential but frankly nobody cares about the marginal effect it has on spermatozoa survival. Prostatic fluid also makes the vagina slightly less hostile for sperm, but in exchange for this meagre benefit men literally lose the ability to pee. A man might have a few kids but urinates perhaps 200,000 times in his life, so I am baffled why this frequent act is deemed less important.

Then we must come to prostate cancer, which is a risk factor for almost every man over a certain age. The only reason we don't just whip the pointless lump out is literally because it's wrapped around vital pipes. My last word on the prostate is that it is a somewhat desperate structure trying to remain at the centre of attention like some narcissistic fungus. So, should men find themselves concerned about what's going on down there in any shape or form, an early check-in with the doctor could make be the difference between life and death.

Dick move

When it comes to the penis – a conduit for both urine and semen – the predilection for the body to combine functions into a biological multi-adaptor is in full effect. Although it might be fun to play with, the delicate structure of the penis leaves it open to catastrophe. Sex is a case in point, as the act requires the male member to be erect. And while the schnozwangler doesn't have a bone, it can still fracture.

The two main components of spongy tissue inside a penis are called the corpora cavernosa. These are enveloped by a fibrous tissue known as the tunica albuginea. It's effectively a membrane that keeps the blood contained within so the penis doesn't just revert to a blood-filled soggy noodle. However, when the penis becomes erect, the tunica also becomes rigid, very thin and – worryingly – quite breakable. The fact is an erect penis can only withstand so much bend before structural failure, and this can occur during vigorous, gymnastic or unsynchronised sex. Once this threshold is crossed, the tunica albuginea can tear, exposing the corpus cavernosa and allowing blood to escape. This is a surgical emergency as much as the stuff of nightmares.

The breaking of a penis is often associated with a popping sound and results in something known as an aubergine (or eggplant) deformity. This is down to the fact that the penis quickly becomes blackish-purple and swollen like the vegetable in question. Unsurprisingly, it's also accompanied by detumescence, in which the hard pork sword becomes a soggy hot dog. Please do not look up aubergine or eggplant deformity.

VAGINAL VENTURES AND INCUBATOR ISSUES

Playgrounds and sewage pipes

If you were to build an amusement park next to a waste disposal centre, eyebrows would be raised. In the same way, the close approximation of the female genitals to the rectum should have drawn attention from Health & Safety at the planning stage, not to mention Sales & Marketing. Given the hygiene considerations at play, it has been the root cause of various ailments, from urinary tracts infections to itchy bottoms.

I would admit that the body offers few alternative sites, at least not without triggering local protests. Frankly, if the anus was located close to the mouth we'd most likely prefer to starve ourselves to death. So, having the back passage close to the genitals, for men as well as women, is perhaps the least bad option. Even so, one would think a bigger gap might have been more appropriate.

The female genitals make things all the more complicated by performing multiple roles. The entrance to the vaginal and urethral pipes are located inside the vulva, in closer proximity to each other than they are to the anus, but combining to form a kind of triangle of potential bacteria displacement and the grief of UTIs (urinary tract infections) and STIs (sexually transmitted infections).

In addition to intercourse and urination, women deploy this area to push out newborn babies. This issue is further compounded by the fact that the female urethra is significantly shorter than the male edition, thus increasing infection risk significantly. The length of the female urethra is approximately 4cm in comparison to the generous 20cm male urethra, which makes any kind of infection quick to reach the bladder. E Coli (Escherichia coli) is a particularly bothersome bug which is responsible for the vast majority of UTIs. It's also a common cause of violent, exorcistic diarrhoea.

Bacteria can commandeer and enter the female urinary tract via several ingenious ways; one is through the act of sex but they can also be ushered in through wiping from back to front after urination and having a bowel motion. I maintain that one of the most important things we fail to teach girls in sexual health is the art of wiping from front to back after going to the toilet.

For both sexes, UTIs don't merely involve the bladder. They can progress retrograde and involve the kidneys too. Typically, telltale signs include a burning sensation when you pee; this is due to activation of TRPV1 receptors by the invading bacteria, which are also triggered by capsaicin in spicy foods. So, your burn is really a burn! Other symptoms include a dull pressure below your belly button – which is where your bladder is located – increased peeing frequency and often blood in the urine as well as an offensive smell. If your body fails to control the bacteria and they march into your kidneys, symptoms can be far more serious and systemic. We're talking about everything from shivers to fevers, vomiting and generally feeling like you've been blitzed by a bus load of microbes.

Save yourself

Men and women may not always be able to prevent UTIs, but there are measures you can take to reduce the risk of this pesky condition. Arguably, a basic and important note here is not to ignore symptoms assuming they will go away. A bacterial urine infection is highly likely to continue to get worse without antibiotics. Untreated, it could even land you in a less than comfortable hospital bed, possibly with a plastic tube shoved into the pipe causing the problem in the first place.

I like to think of the urethra as a ladder that the bacteria can use to make their assault on your waterworks system and beyond. In an attempt to win the battle before it is fought, there is some anecdotal evidence to suggest that staying hydrated helps. This encourages you to pee regularly and flush out any bacteria attempting to slip in unnoticed. This flushing to irrigate the pipes may also work wonders before and after sexual intercourse. In effect it reduces the bacterial load along with the chances of any of them finding themselves somewhere they don't belong.

My final point might be a controversial one – particularly as there is an entire pseudoscientific industry geared towards this – but I would recommend that women avoid douching and inserting so called 'feminine hygiene products' in there. Like the ear, the vagina is a self-sufficient and self-cleaning apparatus with its own unique ecosystem of microbes, bacteria and delicately maintained pH balance. Any foreign substances, including excessive amount of water and irrigation, disrupt the flora and fauna housed within the vagina leading to yeast infections and other ailments.

Ode to the uterus

I want to pay tribute to the uterus; a 3D printer that no one ordered. As a non-owner, however, I must confess that I'm in awe of this function. The uterus has produced every single human to have ever lived, but I think it would be fair to say that the monthly maintenance cycle leaves a little bit to be desired.

Like a rogue sleeper cell/special agent, the uterus is chilled out for 95 per cent of the time. Once in a while it grows a new human along with another absolute dynamite organ, the placenta. I know guys like to think they are the only ones with an organ that can get bigger when called upon but the uterus goes from the size of a pear to the size of a football. Fashioned from pure muscle, it's so strong that it pushes the aforementioned stupidly big-headed small person out through that narrow birth canal. In serving as the incubation chamber for every human that has ever lived, the uterus is worthy of several accolades, even if it does tend to lose the plot every month.

What is the purpose of periods?

It's common for people to settle for the fact that the menstrual cycle is the means by which the female body prepares for pregnancy, but it's a lot more complicated than that. So, gather round and let's hear the extraordinary tale of the period.

Most mammals don't menstruate. It's the preserve of higher primates. What's more, the human female menstruates more than any other creature. From an evolutionary point of view, it's hard to ignore the considerations packaged in with the central purpose. It could be said to be a waste of important nutrients, often very painful and an easy clue to nearby predators. So, why do other mammals that menstruate manage to get through pregnancy with relative ease while dropping litters of dozens and more? Why are humans the tortured ones?

It all comes down to the weird organ called the placenta.

Human females, along with monkeys, rabbits, apes, rats and mice, have something that most mammals don't: a hemochorial placenta. During pregnancy, it forms and burrows deep into the thick layer of endometrial tissue to plug into the mother's blood supply. There, this uncompromising foetal representative siphons off enough blood to supply the greedy growing embryo. At the same time, it keeps the maternal arteries pumped full of chemicals and hormones that prevent them from constricting and reducing the flow of blood. This gives the placenta near unrestricted access to the mother's blood supply. What does all this have to do with menstruation? Patience, padawan.

Clearly, pregnancy places huge demands on the body, and the hemochorial placenta calls most of the shots. Once it sets in, the mother loses a lot of control over her hormones. She also risks haemorrhage when it becomes detached after delivery. In this view, it makes sense for the body to vet and screen embryos very carefully before they implant, because going through pregnancy with a non-viable foetus isn't worth the risk to life.

Then we come to the endometrium. This isn't a cuddly, warm environment for the delicate embryo to nestle in. It's a tough, hostile testing ground where only the hardiest of embryos can survive. What ensues is a cat-and-mouse game between uterus and embryo. This protects the mother, because the longer she can delay the placenta from accessing the mainframe (the bloodstream), the more time she has to determine whether the embryo is viable. Meantime, the embryo wants to unroll its placenta as quickly as possible to tap into the rich blood supply and increase the potential mother's stake in its survival. As a result, the endometrium becomes increasingly thicker; in response the foetal placenta becomes more invasive and aggressive.

As a monthly solution, when the body determines that a healthy pregnancy isn't on the cards, it sloughs off the entire surface lining of the endometrium. It's essentially a form of natural selection that somehow just works, but not without significant downsides such as a risk of menorrhagia (heavy periods) and endometriosis (when tissue similar to that found in the womb lining grows in places like the ovaries, bladder or even the lungs!). These can be so debilitating for sufferers, with their daily routines and lives significantly disrupted.

Even without any associated gynaecological conditions, the uterus during menstruation undergoes one of the most painful biological processes known to humans. This is called ischaemia. When the muscular layer of the uterus has itself in a headlock, it causes compression of the uterine vessels. This results in a temporary cessation of blood flow to these tissues, and is just one of the reasons why periods can be so painful.

The great egg jump

Remember in school biology classes when you were shown a diagram of the uterus, fallopian tubes and ovaries all neatly fixed together like a Lego structure? Well, I hate to break it to you but there is a gap between the ovaries and fallopian tubes. This occurs because they're derived from different tissue types, which means they develop separately. Regardless, the eggs produced in the ovaries must cross a small but treacherous chasm between the ovaries and fallopian tubes. In order to maximise the chances of success, the eggs usually connect with the finger-like tentacles on the end of the fallopian tubes called fimbriae, which sweep them into the tubes towards the ovary.

If a fertilised egg loses its way and doesn't reach the uterus, the most common place it gets stuck or lost is in the fallopian tube where it implants and causes something known as an ectopic pregnancy. Clearly this isn't the appropriate place, and it can result in an agonising gynaecological emergency in which the fallopian tube must be removed.

In the very rare case that a fertilised egg falls into the abdominal cavity, it can be even more catastrophic. There are extremely limited but frightening case reports of a fertilised embryo wandering its way into the liver, a high vascular and blood-rich organ. Suffice to say, the liver is not built to support a pregnancy, and can result in death for the mother.

Stone babies

Stories of ectopic pregnancies – and more specifically abdominal ectopic pregnancies – are understandably tragic and unsettling. It doesn't end there, however. In rare cases, it can result in the creation of a stone baby, or lithopedion.

When a foetus dies during an abdominal pregnancy, and becomes too large for the tissues to be reabsorbed, the body treats it as a potentially harmful foreign substance. In an attempt to protect itself, the body sets about calcifying the foetus. The 'stone baby' that results is often mistaken as a lump that presents no problems. In some cases, they have remained cocooned in the mother's body for years, and sometimes even decades.

ALL ABOUT THE WATERWORKS

Don't hold it in

You've done it on countless occasions. Indeed, healthcare workers the world over are as guilty of this as I am, but it's not good for a variety of reasons. Resisting the urge to urinate is thankfully quite easily done, and yet it's far better for your body to just answer that call when it comes.

Contrary to popular belief, your bladder and urine is not sterile. It's a dark cavern filled with all sorts of funky fungi, bacteria, viruses, dead cell and tissue fragments; if these substances are allowed to fester, they provide a fertile ground for bacteria to multiply and cause you misery down the line.

So, the next time you're at the cinema and feel the urge, don't be tempted to wait until the credits roll. Peeing is a vital task. Your kidneys filter out excess salt, water and waste from your blood. They then distils it into urine, which ends up in your bladder via the ureter. Your bladder, the ingenious coin purse that holds all the golden pennies you will eventually spend, has a storage capacity of around 500–700ml (about 2 cups of water). Typically, you'll feel an urge to relieve yourself when the 300ml threshold is hit.

Just like the art of emptying your bowels, the expulsion of liquid gold is (mostly) a precise and voluntary exercise in symphonic coordination. It's a collaboration between the brain centre that regulates urination, the detrusor muscle of the bladder, the internal and external urethral sphincters and finally some assistance from the pelvic floor muscles. When your bladder fills up with liquid, stretch signals are sent to the brain telling you it's time to pee. In response, your brain communicates back to your bladder to give the green light to open the floodgates or hold on. This is a key step, otherwise things could get messy.

Interesting, for mammals over 1kg, the duration of urination across most species is relatively consistent with an average of 21 seconds. Despite significant differences in bladder volumes in larger creatures, it seems the duration is industry standard. This is thought to be due to an increased urethral length of larger animals and hence an increased amplified flow rate due to gravity.

If you make a habit of regularly holding in your pee and ignoring the reflexive contraction signals, your bladder can stretch beyond a reasonable level to hold even more urine. As superpowers go, this is high up on my list. However, while occasional bladder holding is harmless, regular attempts isn't always a good thing. In some cases, it can weaken the bladder muscles and dampen down the stretch signals. Ultimately, this can lead to some loss in bladder recoil, as well as a reduction in stretch intensity, which is required to tell you about pee volume. As a result, it makes it more difficult for you to release pee normally. In some cases, this over-stretched bladder might end up requiring a catheter to aid in urination.

There exists a far more visceral fate from holding in your pee too much, and that's a burst bladder. Thankfully this worst-case eventuality is incredibly rare. The chances of being beset by an exploded bladder is very low but never zero. When a bladder bursts, the abdominal cavity is quickly filled with urine, requiring immediate emergency surgery.

When it comes to delaying a wee, you're more likely to wet yourself than suffer from a burst bladder. Just be aware that if you're able to resist what is largely an involuntary opening of the floodgates, there is always a chance that the structure could fail, and that carries a significant risk of death. Be warned.

While your bladder may be able to withstand stubbornness on your part when it comes to peeing, repeatedly holding on is more likely to result in incontinence. This is down to a weakening of the pelvic floor muscles, the ones which form a sling around your pelvic organs and which form part of your core muscles. Urinary incontinence is also common in women after childbirth or people who have had major pelvic surgery who then find themselves leaking some urine after a sneeze, cough or even a laugh. Unfortunately, age catches up with us all, which means those taught pelvic floor muscles can become slack and we're back to the risk of wetting our pants as we did as small children.

In addition to possibly compromising the pelvic floor muscles, you might also stretch and weaken the external urethral sphincters. These muscular gatekeepers control the flow of pee; squeeze them and you keep the taps off, relax them and they spin open. Overstretching them can cause you to lose control. It usually occurs only with chronic pee retention, but can result in socially awkward experiences where unexpected leakage ensues.

Save yourself

Mercifully, you can fight the ravages of time by including pelvic floor muscle exercises into your daily routine. We're talking about your core muscles here, which can be activated by imagining that you're trying to hold in a pee or a poo for a few seconds. Remember, this is a simulation to strengthen muscles, which will respond positively by repeating the exercise ten to fifteen times in a daily session. So, if you actually need to go then don't resist the call of nature.

Just in case

You will probably start to despise me after this next bit. Having extolled the virtues of not holding in your pee all the time by means of scare tactics, I'm now going to explain why you should stop doing the 'just in case' piss.

Let me set the scene: you're lying in bed, enjoying the luxury of peak comfort. Suddenly, you convince yourself that you need to make a liquid deposit in the porcelain bank. You ignore this though and try to get back to sleep, only to find yourself plagued by anxiety about wetting the bed. Giving in, you trudge to the toilet for the 'just-in-case' urination, knowing full well it won't be your last one for the night.

Your bladder is a creature of comfort; a petulant child who you indulge at their slightest urge to go to the toilet. Just like any good parent, sometimes you must remind it who sets the rules.

It's prudent to do a 'safety wee' before a long journey, of course, and every once in a while it's no big deal. A routine pitstop when you don't really need one means your bladder fails to fill to full capacity when you use it. In effect, you're setting the threshold to trigger the pee urge at a low bar, so you end up feeling the urge more frequently. In some cases, this causes your bladder to shrink, not anatomically but functionally to accommodate the lower fill-up volumes, thus limiting its capacity when there really was no need to do so. The end result is a nasty snowball effect that can leave you feeling as if your bladder is full when in reality there's plenty of room in the tank.

Save yourself

If you suffer from a frequent need to pee, or any hint of urinary incontinence, your bladder could well be a candidate for retraining. This is not a rigorous ab-shredding type workout but a form of behaviour therapy that helps you regain control of your rogue organ. Taking up to three months or more, it essentially encourages you to gradually increase your bladder capacity to normal levels and then train it to hold in urine for longer periods of time.

You might think it would be less hassle to simply drink less so you don't have to go to the toilet as much. This is an unwise plan. Apart from risking kidney stones, if you restrict your fluid intake you end up with highly concentrated urine in the bladder. This can act as an irritant, which provokes yet more urgency.

Hosepipe pressures

Peeing is an art. When mastered, it should occur when nature calls without a second thought. However, the fly in the soup is that the pelvic floor muscles and the bladder sometimes malfunction, particularly when not used properly. As a result, peeing becomes less of an art and more homework.

Have you ever forced out your urine? Bearing down to squeeze out the pee? You shouldn't. The bladder works and empties best when the pelvic floor muscles and abdominal muscles are slightly relaxed. When you tense your abs and squeeze the pelvic floor muscles during the act of a pee, you're confusing the natural order of things and conditioning your brain to tense the pelvic floor muscles when in fact they should be relaxed. When contracted, the pressure around the bladder neck and urethra is elevated. This limits the full emptying of your bladder, which I've already expressed is bad.

If you continue to regularly force out urine you may develop a staccato stop-start flow pattern because your poor pelvic floor muscles are confused. Furthermore, if you're a dude then I'm sorry to tell say you have a prostate problem. Difficulty urinating or having to squeeze it out could be a symptom of something like benign prostatic hyperplasia, a non-cancerous prostate enlargement. Flow issues could also be down to nerve-issues, an effect of medication or a urine infection. Ultimately, if you're plagued by poor flow and difficulty urinating, check in with a doctor.

Save yourself

This is the part where I tell you the 'healthy' way to pee. Contrary to popular opinion, sitting down to pee provides optimal flow dynamics for both women AND men. There is less pressure on your core, which means your pelvic floor is relaxed.

While sitting should be encouraged, I would avoid squatting or hovering over toilets. It is very unlikely you can get an STD from a public toilet, but if you're struggling to settle over a chipped, still-warm loo seat then cover it with paper first. Hovering over the loo just raises the risk of incomplete bladder emptying due to tightened pelvic floor muscles.

If you are in a rush and need to strain to make it quick, make sure you wait until your stream has started before squeezing. Tightening up before you've begun risks shutting off the valves that allows urine to exit the body. Pee patience will aways pay off.

Do you have the stones?

Your body has a penchant for stones, from gallstones to salivary stones and even navel stones (attractively created by a massing of skin oil, hair and dead skin, and which can prove stubborn to remove from the folds of your belly button). More often than not, this quirk of your body provides you with no material benefit but simply despair, pain and hopelessness.

Kidney stones, those worthless gems of the abdomen, are formed when waste products from the blood crystallise over time. In kidneys that aren't being as challenged as they should be by a regular intake of fluid, phosphate, oxalate, calcium and cystine can combine and harden into a lump. This can subsequently become lodged in the crenulations and crevices of your water pipes, from your kidneys to your ureters to the bladder. Kidney stones are a bit of misnomer most of the time. The most painful variety that patients present to the hospital are found in the ureters, the pipes the carry urine from the kidney to the bladder. These notoriously thin pipes are excellent at holding grudges and, as it turns out, stones too when you don't water yourself enough.

The reason why kidney stones that catch in the ureter are so painful is a no-brainer; why would a sharp, spiky rock stuck in tight, soft squishy tubing hurt slightly? A stone in the pee pipe also blocks the flow of urine from the kidney. This causes the walls of the ureter to stretch like a balloon, which is excruciating.

If you've had one of these malicious crystals lurking in your belly, you will remember it until the day you leave your corporeal form. Sadly, for most people, a kidney stone isn't just a whirlwind unromantic affair. It's a toxic ex that can reappear in your life at the most inopportune of times. There might not be much you can do to eliminate the risk of kidney stones altogether but there are some risk-reducing measures you can take.

Save yourself

It isn't rocket science, or even neuroscience for that matter, but the simplest way to avoid most cases of kidney stones from forming is by staying hydrated. While I don't recommend you drink a generic pre-set amount of water, make sure your urine appears straw-coloured (not dark yellow), your lips and mouth don't feel dry, your skin feels plump and you don't feel thirsty (and if exercising or an excessively hot day, drink a bit extra to be on the safe side). Water dilutes the urine, which can prevent urinary chemicals from crystallising. It's also worth noting that the citrate in beverages with a lemon content may also have a role in helping to prevent stone formation.

I mentioned that oxalate is involved in kidney stone formation; to that end eating calcium-rich foods such as dairy, bread and vegetables is key. This enables calcium to bind to oxalate in your guts, which reduces the amount that is processed and excreted by the kidneys. Ultimately, this helps to lower the levels of oxalate in the urine and cuts down the chances of it binding to the urinary calcium that leads to painful stones. In the same way, keeping salt intake to a minimum can also help you to avoid the problem from forming in the first place.

If you consume excessive amounts of animal protein, and have had stones in the past, you might want to cut down on your red meat intake. Guzzling lots of pork and beef elevates your uric acid levels, which can culminate in a higher risk of stones. Additionally, an excessively high protein diet can reduce those all-important citrate levels. You needn't abstain from red meat and high protein intakes altogether, but if you are prone to stones then aim to limit yourself to no more than 70g of red meat a day.

[Half Page Illustration To Come]

Health Hack

Peeing on a regular basis, and checking that it's straw-coloured or even clear, is a simple way to check you're properly hydrated. An even quicker method, which doesn't involve a trip to the toilet, is to pinch the skin over any finger joint for a second or so.

This is known as the Skin Turgor Test. The more hydrated you are, the more elastic your skin will be, which means it'll swiftly settle back into shape.

If it takes a while, you'd be wise to sip a glass of water to top up your fluid intake.

12. Eyes Wide Shut

HOW SLEEP CAN SLAY YOU

TOWARDS THE END of my first year as a doctor, the accumulative fatigue of stressful shifts combined with the looming anxiety of postgraduate surgical exams turned me into an accidental 3am riser. My 'sleep', if you could dare to call it that, was a glorified elongated nap punctuated with awakenings. For weeks, I was in denial. I couldn't possibly have insomnia, I told myself. That just wasn't me.

I could complain about the terrible shift patterns and work commitments spilling into my home life, but frankly I didn't take sleep seriously. I saw it as a task that needed to be checked off at the end of the day. My mindset was 'I can sleep when I'm dead.' It was one of those invincible doctor mantras with no grounding in science, because the fact is poor sleep ushers you towards an early grave. Reminding myself of this, it took me months of dedicated 'sleep work' to figure out what I was doing wrong and ultimately rectify my litany of errors.

THE SHORTCOMINGS OF SLEEP

Simply put, sleep is the foundation of all facets of health – both mental and physical. It underpins all forms of cognitive and physical performance. Sleep even reaches beyond its assigned remit and controls things like your immune system, wound healing, skin health and your appearance. Unfortunately, your body's battery capacity is about as limited as most smartphones. It needs regular charging, which occurs during sleep, because if left to run empty it can result in calamitous consequences.

Slave to the rhythm

You might think that you eat when hungry, drink when thirsty and sleep when you feel tired. You have control over these things, right? While you may appear to have the illusion of ample choice here, this is a mere pretence. If your material devices were extracted and you lived in a world bereft of artificial lights, alarm clocks and rigidly structured work hours then your sleep, thirst, hunger and various other biological calls would be decided not by you, but by your tyrannical time lord, the internal biological clock – also known as the suprachiasmatic nucleus.

This small but dense collection of 20,000 neurons deep inside your brain is the pacemaker of your life. It dictates not just your physical behaviour but also the sway of your mood and emotion on a daily basis. This internal metronome is highly sensitive to temperature, darkness and light cues, and yet the real control monitor lies deep within your brain. This is the device that instructs you to sleep and wake up. In fact, among many other functions, it also tells your body when to release hormones and even adjust your body temperature.

Everything from your heartbeat to your bowel motions is influenced by the time of day. The rotation of the earth on its axis creates these daily cycles of light, temperature and other things to which your biological processes are enslaved. In fact, all the cells in your body contain little timepieces that are governed by the grandfather clock in your brain. This operates on a 24-hour cycle called the circadian rhythm. Any significant disruption to it can even impact on your lifespan. You only have to try going without sleep for a week to recognise that ignoring it might not be that good for you.

Despite the fact that evolution and life has enslaved you to the circadian rhythm for good reason, you and your body take every opportunity to rebel against it. You guzzle coffee to fight drowsiness, blast the radio and then roll down the windows to stay focused when in fact you should be asleep. Thanks to your prefrontal cortex, which convinces you that you know best, you'll try every trick in the book to give the sandman the slip. No matter how hard you fight, however, it is a pyrrhic victory. You can win, but you pay a heavy price. Disruption to your circadian rhythm impacts not just sleep but also your metabolic function and mood, your body's stress response and various hormones that govern appetite, energy, thyroid function and beyond.

Light cycling

Increasingly we seek out dark spaces. By choice, you tuck yourself away at home, in offices and in shopping malls, relinquishing the outside like troglodytes. In doing so deprive yourself of the very thing that helps you to sync your daily rhythm: sunlight.

For over a century we've known about the two main light receptors in the retina, the rods and cones. It's only recently, however, that we've stumbled upon the fact that the eye contains a third light sensor. This one is non-visual, but is vital in maintaining your sleep–wake cycle. Without it, you would drift increasingly out of sync with time, and effectively your life would become a mess. This means you can be visually blind and yet your eyes still have the ability to set your internal clock. Unfortunately, some people who have their eyes removed prophylactically by ophthalmologists may also find themselves unwittingly cast into a world of perpetual jet lag.

Morning glory

For millennia, human sleep and wake patterns were delicately in tune with the natural cycles of dark and light. Your 24-hour body clock evolved in an era before mobile phone screens, TVs, bedroom lamps and streetlights. It was rigged to keep you synched by the rise and fall of the sun. Now we live in an age of technology. For all the advantages this brings, it also carries an unwelcome level of artificial light disruption. As a result, your sleep health suffers.

In order to get things back on track, I want to talk about the first thing you absolutely need to do in the morning. This might seem strange for a chapter about sleep, but indulge me. One of the main triggers that wakes you up is a rise in body temperature along with an increase in the production of a hormone called cortisol. As it's often described as a 'stress' hormone, we often wrongly demonise cortisol and seek to avoid it. The fact is that when it's released in specific amounts at certain times – such as when you wake up – cortisol allows you to focus mentally, increase your metabolism and fully shake off the remaining particles of sleep dust. Light, by this token, is an alertness-boosting agent – like a biological espresso. It's great in the morning but bad news if you're trying to get some shut-eye at night.

Save yourself

A fail-safe means of getting your cortisol hit at the optimum time is by exposing yourself to bright light or sunshine within the first hour of waking. Even if it's overcast, the UV light still percolates through clouds. This triggers neurons in your eye that signal to the internal body clock (the suprachiasmatic nucleus), and thus causes a surge in cortisol. Not only does this work like an alarm clock for your brain and body, but it also sets in motion a timer for you to fall asleep later that night. Additionally, it will suppress the hormone melatonin while washing out the adenosine system, both of which can make you tired at a time when you need to be seizing the day.

Ultimately, viewing morning light not only provides you with the most powerful biological stimulus to wake up in the morning, but it also has a powerful impact on your ability to fall and stay asleep at night.

SLEEP IS A MAGIC NUMBER

Like a rapidly draining rechargeable battery, the human body needs to be plugged into the sleep mains to renew its energy reserves.

Do you need seven hours sleep? Eight hours? Is there a case to go to nine? Unfortunately, there is no black and white answer. At its most reductive level, you need enough sleep to allow you to wake up feeling refreshed and alert. Multiple factors come into play here, such as your age, genetics and environment. In fact, 'normal' sleep can vary from four hours to eleven, but on average most people are somewhere between seven and eight. Some even have a genetic variant, the DEC-2 gene mutation, which allows them to get away with sleeping just four or five hours a night while retaining the cognitive performance of someone who has slept much longer.

Sleeping in segments

In order to work out how much downtime you need, it's worth having a basic understanding of what goes on during sleep. This begins by recognising that the brain doesn't shut down as you're snoring – it's highly active during this process. There are four stages of sleep to consider, and the key to achieving body and mind restoration lies in a delicate balancing of them all. Within each stage, you can undergo one of two essential phases: REM (rapid eye movement), in which the brain is relatively active and dreams can take place, and the deeper, more restorative sleep that takes place called non-REM (NREM).

* Stage 1 is NREM and lasts up to 10 minutes as your body begins to relax; at this stage you can be easily aroused.

* Stage 2 is NREM and lasts slightly longer, up to 25 minutes. Your heart rate progressively slows but this is still considered a light sleep.

* Stage 3 is NREM and lasts up to 40 minutes. It's a key deep sleep phase (slow wave sleep) that is required to repair your body and is a determinant in how alert and refreshed you will be when you wake up.

* Stage 4 begins with the first REM phase. It's another deep stage but your brain is still highly active – similar to your waking hours.

It is in this REM stage that you can be assaulted by sleepwalking, sleeptalking and vivid nightmares and dreams.

These four cycles take around ninety minutes to complete, and one night's sleep will see you go through up to four or five cycles. As you progress through the cycles, the proportion of NREM to REM changes. The early part of the night is dominated by the deeper, more restorative NREM sleep. As you get towards daybreak so your REM sleep becomes predominant. Regardless of what time you choose to go to bed, you will always shift from NREM to REM sleep, and this happens at specific parts of the night according to your circadian rhythm. So, if you go to bed much later than usual your sleep will be more REM heavy. With less of the deeper NREM sleep, chances are you'll wake up feeling groggy. You only have yourself to blame, of course. Unless you're a shift worker.

Save yourself

If you find that you're being snatched awake by your alarm, it's worth reviewing your sleep routine. Either you're not getting enough, or you're ignoring a moment some time before the alarm goes off when your body is ready to rise. As a result, you plunge into another sleep cycle that's destined to be cut short. This can be particularly upsetting if you happen to be in an NREM cycle at the time, because you'd never naturally wake from this deep sleep phase. The alarm clock doesn't care, however, and could disrupt this crucial deep sleep stage in which the brain is resting and sorting out its household chores. If you are woken up from this stage, you'll feel groggy and heavy, as if you have a hangover – this is sleep inertia, as the hormones that promote alertness haven't reached their zenith yet. Your brain has essentially been jump-started to a state of wakefulness instead of a gradual rise. This shock to the system triggers a stress response that can mean you start your day with a high heart rate and blood pressure.

The simplest way of determining how much sleep your body needs is to establish your desired wake up time and then work backwards. The aim is to wake up naturally just before your alarm, and you can achieve this with some experimentation by adjusting your sleep time by going to bed earlier or later. Once you've established a healthy sleep pattern, however, try not to undermine it with weekend lie-ins. Your circadian rhythm doesn't recognise Sundays are a day off, which means sleeping until mid-morning will cause disruption down the line. Essentially, your body anticipates its daily actions based on routine. It's attempting to maintain a semblance of efficiency through rigid timing, from metabolism to organ function and even gene expression.

Ultimately, if you've nailed a good sleep pattern then you won't even need an alarm. For one thing, your body hates the damned things. It's stressful on a biological level and highly jarring. In a bid to avoid being blasted out of bed on a regular basis, your body increases the protein which regulates your sleep–wake cycle to give you a head start on the waking up process. This can be so precise that you might find your eyelids opening minutes or even seconds before your alarm sounds. If so, take it as a sign that your sleep routine is on track.

What goes on during sleep?

In a deep sleep, your subconscious brain consolidates a flurry of fleeting thoughts into long-term memories. Alongside this filing action, a cerebral cleansing process takes place to wash the filth away – both literally and metaphysically. During the day, your brain has accumulated an assortment of misshapen protein and trash. In sleep, out of hours, an undulating wave of cerebrospinal fluid washes it away into the in-house waste disposal unit, the glymphatic system. If left to build up, such detritus can contribute to neurodegenerative diseases like dementia.

Sleep has evolved because it offers multiple benefits for mind and body. It is the point in the day where the production of growth hormones reaches its peak and stimulates the regeneration of damaged tissue. It plays a vital role in boosting your immune system, memory consolidation and emotional regulation.

Less sleep means more of the stress hormone cortisol. This raises the flow of blood to the skin surface causing puffy, dark circles around the thin skin under the eyes. Your blood glucose metabolism is also affected, which increases your risk of metabolic issues, insulin resistance and chronic heart disease.

The snag with sleep is that your body requires you to be submerged into a state of suspended animation with no vigilance detection system in place. That makes you a ready meal for a prowling tiger. At the same time, you are unable to eat, drink or reproduce; the very human things you like to do that are also key for survival. If sleep didn't serve a vital function it would be the biggest mistake evolution made. Clearly the multitude of benefits it offers make it worth the risk of lying immobile in the darkness of the night.

What happens if you don't sleep enough?

In 1963, two teenage boys attempted to stay awake for as long possible. In a bid to win a local science competition, Randy Gardner and Bruce McAllister aimed to experience the effects of sleep deprivation on cognitive and physical performance. The two lads flipped a coin to determine the roles of guinea pig and observer. Randy lost.

There is only one reason why this story made it into the annals of bizarre medical history, and that's because it was covered by the local media. As a result, Randy's planned bid came to the attention of Stanford University sleep researcher Dr William Dement.

Until that time, scientific experiments on sleep deprivation had resulted in paranoia, emotional lability (rapid changes in mood) and various other issues. Death was also a side effect not to be disregarded, and so it came as some relief to the boys when Dement offered to supervise the experiment, along with an officer from the US Navy Neuropsychiatric Research Unit.

To keep Randy stimulated, the team would play pinball and basketball with him, stop him from lying down and even keep him talking when in the toilet to avoid any sneaky naps. The first 24 hours went by smoothly. Day two however, saw Randy experience difficulty identifying objects with his sense of touch. On day three he became irritable and found it difficult to enunciate certain words. Day four was peppered with memory lapses and the occasional hallucination. The hallucinations then grew in intensity and frequency on day five.

Over the following six days, Randy's mood slumped. His speech began to slow and slur; often leaving sentences half complete. He was, however, still able to play table tennis. At the end of the experiment, and a total of 264.4 hours spent awake, Randy was expressionless and speaking in monotone, and yet appeared free from major ill effects. He had a new world record.

The experiment suggested that during the course of his marathon wake time, parts of his brain had essentially switched to sleep mode. Other have since broken this world record, although it's worth noting that the Guinness World Records have stopped accepting attempts for this highly dangerous activity.

Sleep scheduling

It's often difficult to determine whether a disrupted internal clock leads to health problems or vice versa. Either way, keeping your body's daily cycle on an even platform might be one of the best zero-cost acts you can do for overall health. The idea that you have a biological clock may seem like just another funny metaphor but the truth is your body demands it runs like a Swiss watch.

If you wake up at 6am every morning, and go to bed at 10pm at night, your body becomes used to this sleeping pattern. It means it knows exactly when to release certain hormones like melatonin that make you sleepy. If you mess with that sleeping pattern and stay out until 1am, your body reads the delay as a threat. So, rather than power you down, the brain releases stress hormones to help you stay alert. Your body is just trying to survive, but it ends up ruining your sleep quality and duration. By respecting your circadian rhythm as realistically as you can, sleep becomes a certainty rather than a surprise.

Working 9–5

Like a vast chunk of the world, if you work a regular day job, struggle to get up in the morning and feel yourself sinking in energy levels in the afternoon then you can thank Henry Ford, the founder of the Ford Motor Company. In the 1920s, Ford instilled the 9–5 practice to deliver ultra-efficient production lines in his factories. Over a hundred years later, thanks to a surprise pandemic that made it a necessity to work from home, we are increasingly questioning the sanity of rigid working hours.

This is especially highlighted when you take into account your body's specific inclinations to be sluggish or energetic at given times of the day. Biologically speaking, different people have different hormones with unique release schedules. They also experience temperature fluctuations at different times. I despised early starts for most of my life. My dad used to have to drag me out of bed for 7am Sunday swimming lessons with my militant swim coach, and then again on weekday mornings for early school starts. Every time, I'd dress in the half-light with my head throbbing and my stomach contorting with nausea. This inclination to be asleep (or wide awake) at a certain time of day is known as a chronotype. It's largely shaped by your genetic and clock genes, and governs many aspects of your physiology.

Society isn't neatly split into morning larks and night owls, however. There is an entire spectrum of diurnal preferences with the majority of people in the middle leaning more towards one direction or the other.

The point in the night at which half your sleep is done is an indication to your chronotype. It's an important factor, determining how your specific biological clock can influence your daily behaviours. For example, early risers (morning larks) may feel more energised and active in the morning but tired in the later afternoon and early evening. Then you have late chronotypes (night owls) who feel tired in the morning but come alive with energy in the evening. There are also several other versions of these chronotypes that lie somewhere in the middle.

Critically, your chronotype determines when melatonin is released into the body system, which determines your sleep levels and sleep–wake cycle. It matters because typically 'night owls' are viewed as lazy in modern society, in that we tend to take a dim view of late risers. These poor souls subsequently struggle to get the adequate sleep by defying the forces of their biology to hold a 9–5 job. It's no surprise that night owls have a higher risk of health issues if faced with this conundrum.

It's worth noting that your biological response to the passage of time is not immutable. Most people have a morning chronotype when young before gradually donning the cape of a more night-owlish chronotype during adolescence. They may even go through a phase of staying up vampirically late before returning to an earlier rising pattern by old age. By then, that early night comes as a blessed relief.

Just to flatter you further when it comes to being unique, your body clock is custom-built. There is no dormitory that can house people who share exactly the same circadian rhythm. Everyone ticks slightly out of time from each other. Why? One sentinel hypothesis suggests it might serve some ancestral evolutionary purpose. Early human tribes may have benefited from some members staggering their sleep schedules so someone was always at hand to watch for prowling predators. Eventually, the rise of agriculture and the need to use morning hours for productivity meant night owls were relegated to the lower ranks of society. So, rather than perish they were forced to adapt and then live with the health consequences.

Save yourself

Attractively, after a good night's sleep you can still wake up feeling as dried out as a packet of noodles. Although your body has deployed certain safeguards to prevent dangerous levels of dehydration by powering down metabolism, raising the levels of anti-diuretic hormone so you retain as much water as possible, and even dropping your core body temperature, mild dehydration after a night supine (or curled up in a ball) is inevitable. Even this mild dehydration is enough to impact your alertness, focus and mood in the morning. To offset this mental zombification, drink a large glass of water in the morning to refuel your tank.

Ideally, I would recommend reaching for the glass before your mobile phone. Odds suggest that you are guilty of checking it as soon as you prise open your eyelids. From emails to social media and breaking news, you are overwhelmed with distraction, stress and notifications before you're fully up and running.

Prior to waking your brain emerges from the delta wave pattern of deep sleep to the lighter sleep of theta waves. On surfacing, your brain transitions to the alpha waves that will see you through the day, but what it doesn't need to know in that gentle adjustment period is how many overnight likes your last kitten post has picked up. This stuff can wait, and your brain will thank you for it. Exposing yourself to the micro-stresses that will no doubt dominate your day just triggers stress responses. Realistically, for the sake of your well-being, there are very few things that can't be postponed for at least thirty minutes after waking. In that time, for example, you could enjoy a refreshing glass of water.

In addition to low lubrication, your glucose battery pack will be running on empty. The self-inflicted involuntary fast that you undertake overnight depletes blood sugar levels, leaving you irritable and tired.

This can be rectified with a small portion of fruit, even if you're not a 'breakfast person', to restore energy and promote alertness.

Finally, to counter stiffened limbs and the overnight rust that has accumulated in your joints, some brisk activity like a fast-paced walk or even dynamic stretching will help you to break free of the sleep demons and set you up for the day.

The graveyard shift

An altered biological clock can have more significant ramifications than just making it harder to fall asleep or wake up in the morning. The most extreme effects are seen in night shift workers where day and night are swapped. Studies have yielded information that shift workers like medical professionals, factory workers and flight attendants who hop times zones have a significantly higher risk of various cancers, metabolic disease, mental health problems and even cardiovascular disease. In fact, even small alterations by an hour to your circadian rhythms have shown to be deleterious to health – another reason daylight savings needs to be cancelled.

As a regular night shift worker myself, I can attest to the grim feeling that overcomes my body as I peer into the abyss of dysregulated sleep at 3am on a Thursday morning on shift three out of four. The night shift work encompasses a period of the 24-hour cycle in which your cognitive function and mood are at their lowest point. This occurs between 3 and 5am. After the shift, you force your body to rest in a phase less conducive to sleep, which only worsens fatigue and sleep disturbances. It's a challenge for anyone, and a question of establishing strategies and routines that prove to work for you.

Save yourself

When it comes to working when everyone else is in bed, the first fix begins by minimising your sleep debt before the run of night shifts. Why? Because on that first night chances are you will experience an insatiable sleep hunger and reduced ability to perform to your best abilities. Practically speaking, this can be done by allowing unrestricted, undisturbed sleep on the morning before the night shift. This means no set wake up time and no alarms. Bliss! You can even nap in the afternoon, which helps you hijack the natural 'circadian dip' in energy you experience between 2 and 6pm.

A key pillar in many a shift worker's arsenal is caffeine, a stimulant found in coffee. I for one would advocate against this, however. Why? In the main, if you consume it too late into your shift then it could end up compromising your daytime sleep, which also comes pre-packaged with unyielding light, noise and the fight against your biological clock.

All biological processes are slaves to your circadian rhythm, digestion included. The timing of your insulin and glucose secretion timings, liver function, intestinal motility, bowel function and gastric emptying all decrease during the sleep phase, and will do just that if you're fighting your way through a night shift.

Ultimately, it is impossible to expect your body to become 'used to' working after dark on a short-term basis. Long-haul flight passengers will tell you that it takes a few days to adjust. So, the priority here is to optimise your sleep between shifts to reduce sleep debt and fatigue. Key strategies here include avoiding bright daylight on the journey home by considering sunglasses and creating a dark environment in your bedroom to simulate night during day. Minimising daytime noise by using ear plugs will also help you to reduce sleep disruption.

On completing a night shift period of work, or seeking to reset your body clock after long-haul travel, it's advisable to return to a normalised sleeping pattern as quickly as possible. You can achieve this in two key ways. Firstly, aim to use natural light cues to notify your body clock that the rebellion is over. This might mean stepping outside at sunrise and sunset. In between, consider napping for roughly ninety minutes (one full sleep cycle), which will help to soften the final stretch before bed at a civilised time.

PROBLEMS WITH SLEEP

Parasomnia

During sleep, your body frequently stages a power grab that can force you to perform some peculiar if dangerous acts. Parasomnias are considered to be sleep disorders, and raise questions about whether the sufferer should be considered responsible for actions they've no knowledge of undertaking.

At the benign end of the parasomnia spectrum, you'll find acts such as sleeptalking. Sleepwalking might seem harmless, but carries a significant risk of injury. Contrary to what urban myths you may have heard, it is highly advisable to wake up a sleepwalker to prevent them from clattering down flights of stairs or whatever dangers lie in their path. Sexsomnia sees sufferers performing sex acts in their sleep, and in very rare cases individuals have woken to discover that the bad dream in which they killed someone turned out to be true. While most common parasomnias are harmless, and generally see you mumbling nonsense about crumpets and budgerigars, they demonstrate the thin line between sleep and wakefulness.

In general, parasomnias occur during the REM stage of sleep. During this time, the brain fires signals to your muscles allowing them to enact the movements from your dreams. Fortunately, your brain also has a fail-safe signal to the muscles to prevent you from carrying out actions for real by paralysing most of the muscles in your body. All that's free from this lock are the diaphragm, small muscles in the ear and those that move your eyes. In some of these so-called REM behaviour disorder conditions, the normal paralysis of muscles during REM fails to deploy. As a result, with unrestricted movement of all muscles, the sleeper can become a danger to themselves and others.

Sleep paralysis

Every night, your body undergoes a natural, self-administered anaesthesia. It's intended to keep you safe and sound . . . unless you happen to become aware of what's happened. The first time I experienced sleep paralysis was in the week leading up to my medical school finals. At 2am, my eyes were open but my body was frozen. Whether it was the sheer terror that gripped me, or the effects of the horror movie I'd watched a few hours earlier, I swore that I could see some shapeless figure lurking in the corner of my bedroom. Needless to say it was a deeply disturbing moment, and thankfully sleep reclaimed me for the rest of the night.

Throughout history people have described sleep paralysis as a terrifying experience with references made to a figure, mass, alien or demonic presence sitting on their chest.

You might well have experienced this brain glitch yourself. It's believed that a structure in the brainstem called the pons controls the sleep–wake cycle. It's tasked with sending chemicals and signals to your spinal cord to temporarily paralyse your muscles to stop you acting out your outrageous nightmares and running away from giant balls of cheese.

Unfortunately, should you try to wake up, the pons doesn't always turn off the chemicals that keep your muscles in a state of paralysis. This leaves you awake on some level, still partially in a dream-like state with fantastical visions in your mind. It's just your body can't move, which is as close as you'll get to a nightmare made real.

Sleep apnoea

During sleep, a conflict between neck and throat can lead to snoring. While not everyone suffers from this anatomical roadblock, known as obstructive sleep apnoea, it affects millions of people worldwide, who literally stop breathing at multiple points overnight.

Imagine your throat and upper airways as a pipe that must remain clear of blockages to perform its duties. When you're awake, the pipe is open for access in terms of breathing and swallowing. When you lie down for sleep, the muscles around the piping relax. By extension, the surrounding paraphernalia such as the tongue and soft palate can press down on the tube further and interfere with the flow of air. As a result, the pipe can become blocked.

This design error affects the sufferer, who may experience an unrefreshing, choke-peppered night of sleep, followed by daytime fatigue and mental fog. They are also likely to snore, which is effectively the sound of air attempting to pass the nocturnal blockages. As the cherry on the top, this means anyone within earshot is likely to be deprived of sleep, which can also give rise to symptoms of irritability and unreasonableness.

Obvious snoring culprits include swollen adenoids or tonsils, which can be effectively remedied with a surgical operation. Other causes include excessive weight gain. This can result in excess fat around the throat and chest, leading to restricted breathing, and a solution that lies in a sensible weight loss programme. Inevitably, ageing will play a part in the form of degeneration. When it affects the throat, so the sleep symphony begins.

Structurally, the neck is a poorly conceived construct. It's a room with a mishmash of fixtures and fittings that are tightly stuffed together. In some ways, it's the price you pay for that big brain and sophisticated speech capacity. With little space left, you have to put up with a small oral cavity and a right angle bend in the tongue among other things. Obstructive sleep apnoea is literally and figuratively a pain in the neck, but perhaps also the price you pay for being human.

Save yourself

Sleep is a compulsory part of life. If so inclined, you can only fight it off for so long. Chances are you're happy to go to bed at the end of each day, but how can you be sure that you're about to enjoy a quality sleep with limited risk of nocturnal dramas? It can seem like you're placing yourself in the hands of fate, but in reality there is much you can do to ensure a good night's kip.

• **Be caffeine aware**

The main active ingredient in coffee, caffeine, is the psychoactive drug of choice for many people seeking to boost energy levels. At least that's how caffeine is sold to us. The fact is it should be viewed as an anti-sleep agent rather than a means of increasing alertness. It only appears to give you energy.

From the time you wake up, your body start to accumulate sleep pressure. This is the invisible force that progressively makes you tired throughout the course of the day. Your cells and tissues burn energy in the form of a chemical called adenosine triphosphate (ATP). As you burn up this biological tinder wood, your cells generate adenosine diphosphate (ADP) as a by-product, which then binds to receptors in the brain to make you sleepy.

Caffeine is structurally similar to adenosine. This means it can trick your body by sneaking into the adenosine binding spots. In effect, caffeine interferes with adenosine as it prepares your body for rest and thus prevents you from feeling sleepy. In an act of revenge, adenosine continues to rise and accumulate in the background. So, when the caffeine is eventually metabolised, the adenosine molecules flood their rightful receptors and you feel an overwhelming rush of tiredness. In this light, you can consider caffeine to be a means of pushing sleep back, but ultimately it's a debt you'll have to repay. With interest.

If you must drink caffeine to function, limit your last cup of coffee to no later than 2pm. Anything after that time means you increase the risk of your sleep pressure not adequately building up to drive your body's urge to sleep. This culminates in a vicious cycle of sleep deprivation and poor alertness come morning, which further encourages your need for more coffee throughout the day and so on.

The insidious truth about caffeine is that it is both a tool to remedy the consequence of poor sleep and also to compensate for the awful sleep that caffeine causes. A drug that hides the very problem it helps to create.

• Nail the naps

In the sweltering heat of Mumbai, napping was a mid-afternoon feature of my childhood summers. My fondness for siestas, I later learned, wasn't borne out of the humidity and heat but biology. The human body was designed for such a snooze. It acts as a pressure valve to release the stresses of everyday life. During a nap, your blood pressure and heart rate drop while the immune system consolidates. Research even suggests that naps help boost memory and cognitive performance.

But what is the perfect length for a nap? Is there a biologically advantageous and socially acceptable duration when it comes to getting your head down during the day? There are some appreciable benefits for a twenty-minute nap. This is long enough to allow you to put your brain into reset mode and feel a sense of rejuvenation. Additionally, you are less likely to drift into deeper, slow wave sleep stages that could risk you feeling 'sleep drunk' when you surface.

Longer naps, say ninety minutes (which is my preference) are associated with improvements in performance as well as reduced sleepiness than shorter naps. As you cover one entire sleep cycle, both REM and NREM, you stand to gain improvements in both procedural and emotional memory. The ninety-minute nap technically covers an entire sleep cycle so you should awaken from a lighter stage and thus avoid sleep inertia woes entirely.

As a general rule, assuming you go to bed around 10 or 11pm, limit any naps after 4pm to minimise the hit to your sleep drive.

• Snack sense

The type of food you eat, as well as your meal timings, can influence your quality of sleep. Heavy meals high in fat (like cheese), or large portions eaten close to bedtime, can increase the chances of indigestion and acid reflux. The combination of these things potentially disrupts the sleep cycle, which can result in bad dreams you remember. Based on my personal research into the subject, this is the science behind the bizarre cheese-nightmare association.

Your stomach typically takes around ninety minutes to empty 50 per cent of its contents into the small intestine. Turning in before this time has passed can mean all that gut activity makes it hard to sleep.

• Steer clear of sleeping pills and alcohol

Sleeping pills work by boosting the production of a neurotransmitter called GABA. This can help to quieten down the activity of neurons in the brain. Alcohol has a similar effect. The problem is they're both sedative agents. While they can promote sleep, evidence suggests they may restrict the deeper brain waves seen in the restorative phase, which can contribute to feeling groggy the next morning. It's also worth mentioning that alcohol specifically disrupts REM sleep, which you can add to the list of health risks associated with drinking.

I have prescribed sleeping pills for patients in hospitals, however. Unsurprisingly, with all the shrill beeps and flashing lights at all hours of the night, patient sleep patterns are awful. However, this is a short-term solution for a transient obstacle in most cases. The patient's sleep generally improves once they are discharged and at home. In short, sleeping pills are not a long-term fix; they simply serve to paper over the cracks.

• Wind down

During the day, your body is a car hurtling down the highway. Naturally, when you finish your journey, you gently decelerate before parking. You don't come hurtling in at top speed without significant risk of creating chaos, and the same can be said for your approach to sleep.

In preparation for bedtime, you need to wind down your pulse, blood pressure, breathing and mental state. So, as well as avoiding a late night workout, steer clear of watching adrenaline-fuelled movies with loud noises and stimulating images. A state of anxiety, high energy or racing thoughts is not what you need before bed because it delays your sleep induction (the time it takes for you to fall asleep). Essentially, your brain and body needs that much longer to 'brake' before parking for the night.

Begin the winding-down process mindfully a couple of hours before bed. Reduce the intensity of lights around the house, while minimising screen and TV time. Consider adding some light breathing exercises to consciously slow down your heart and breathing. Reading a book is another effective way to wind down through the gears before easing into the garage of sleep for the night.

• Sleep mode

Not all light is beneficial to your body clock. If you're the type to lie in bed at night with your phone in hand, the light from the screen can be a disruptive influence. This is down to a peculiar asymmetry in your eye and brain biology. Yes, you need lots of photons of light to rouse you in the morning, but at night even a little bit of artificial light can disrupt your circadian rhythm.

There is no hard and fast rule as to when you should leave your phone alone before bed. You're not a child, and I don't wish to prescribe a time that might seem unrealistic or unreasonable. Just be aware that doomscrolling after dark serves to stimulate your brain, and possibly also ramp up your anxiety levels. Factor in all the artificial light that's stimulating your eyeballs and you have a recipe for insomnia.

Ultimately, if you're filled with dread at the thought of putting your phone to sleep an hour before you hope to follow suit, perhaps you need to review your relationship with technology before working to improve your sleep health.

[Half Page Illustration To Come]

Health Hack

We all want a shortcut to a good night's sleep, and a warm shower before bed might just be the key. Paradoxically, the raised temperature of the water serves to cool down your core body temperature and lowers the sleep threshold.

Conversely, a cold shower in the morning can kick-start your day by raising your body temperature and making your more alert. Also cleaner.

13. The War on Bugs

INVESTIGATING THE
IMMUNE SYSTEM

WHAT WE HAVE HERE is the human version of anti-malware. In a biological way, the immune system frequently updates, learns from interactions and auto-renews for the duration of your lifetime. It's a critical piece of code, designed to protect you from all manner of threats. Frustratingly, it also bugs out quite often.

You are part of a sickly species. Humans contract sniffles, colds and flus with far more regularity than other creatures, and that's just the light stuff. You are tormented by a myriad of other illnesses and infections, from violent diarrhoea pouring furiously from your tailpipe to life-threatening allergies that can turn a peanut into a death sentence.

Many of these pathologies that plague you can be directly attributed to mishaps in your immune system. On the whole, it does a decent job. It's just that frequently it takes on more than it can handle. Then, out of nowhere, it can sometimes go rogue and exhibit self-deprecating tendencies.

To be fair, we humans haven't helped our immune systems one iota. We immerse ourselves in densely populated and filthy urban environments. For centuries, we neither understood nor cared for simple hygiene and unwittingly brewed a malevolent cocktail of pathogenic bacteria, vicious viruses and life-sucking parasites. It was only thanks to a few pioneers in the field of hygiene, the invention of the microscope and modern-day plumbing that civilisation even got this far.

The hidden war

At this very moment a conflict is raging, and it's taking place inside your body. An army of microscopic super soldiers wait vigilantly; some patrolling every crevice of your body for danger, others running headfirst into battle, kamikaze-style. These are the goodies. They're on your side, and come under the flag of the immune system. It's been at your service since birth: always there, watching over you. The real question is: who watches the watchmen?

For all its hard work, the immune system has been handed thankless orders. With an army of cells, it strives to keep you safe from a bombardment of bacteria and viruses. Without it, you'd be dead, and yet when it makes the slightest slip and saddles you with a minor cold or pollen allergy, there you go complaining that you're run down as if somehow your internal guard against these things can't be trusted.

With rare exceptions, the immune system never deserts its post. Nevertheless, it's prone to meltdowns and self-destructive behaviours and you are collateral damage. It often misfires and attacks its own cells leading to autoimmune disease. It even overreacts to harmless particles like cat hair, giving rise to potentially life-threatening emergencies. Occasionally it even fails to pick up on abnormal cells that could become cancerous.

Boot camp

Your body is exposed to a vast array of foreign material every day. Even so, we haven't quite figured out how your body determines the difference between harmful external agents and harmless ones. We do know, however, that your immune system undergoes some initial training in the womb and then early childhood.

There is something incredibly sci-fi and slightly dystopian that happens when you're a burgeoning embryonic life form. It's a process known as clonal deletion. Your nascent embryonic immune cells are presented bits of your own foetal proteins. The immune cells that needlessly react to these substances duly fail the test. Without mercy, they are then deleted forever from an immune system intended to attack only foreign invaders.

When you're thrust into this septic world at birth, your immune system has to figure out its actual foes. Oddly enough, the only way it does this is through lived experience. This is why children are constantly sick because they're still amassing their immunity and data on viruses and other bugs.

Locked and loaded

The immune system consists of two arms. The first is called the innate immune response. This is effectively a barrier method which encompasses the skin and the lining of your digestive tract. Both are physical front lines that can stop infective agents from entering your body.

To back up these foot soldiers, your body calls upon state-of-the-art weaponry that operates under the code name of phagocytosis. This is a term used to describe the ingestion of bacteria by cells that can produce interferons – a fancy sci-fi name for a vitally important protein that can limit the replication of virus-infected cells. For all its sophistication, however, the innate immune response employs a scattergun approach to defence. It's a crude, blunt instrument to deal with a perceived threat, resulting in the activation of a rapid inflammatory response with no specific target in mind. So, although pathogens will perish, there's a good chance you can sustain some collateral injury such as generalised inflammation when you pick up a simple infection or suffer from an allergic rash. The innate immune system doesn't always stop such attacks, however, which is why it needs back up.

The adaptive immune response primarily consists of a small, highly trained special ops groups of white blood cells called lymphocytes. These originate from two training camps or 'lineages': B cells and T cells. The

B cell veterans exclusively produce specific immunoglobulins – basically antibodies to detect invading pathogens and nullify the threat. Antibodies can do this by directly binding to invaders and tackling them or binding to toxins that pathogens may produce. Occasionally, they might also flag up any microbes so the innate system patrol unit can destroy them.

As for the T cells, these guys are psychos. We're talking about a group of reckless, kamikaze soldiers that can destroy cancer cells or even virus-infected cells and show no mercy. Additionally, there are helper T cells that can help both B and killer T cells do their job.

The antibodies that are produced by B cells hang around in your bloodstream for years in case a once-repelled enemy mounts another attack. While most of the killer T cells die off once their contract is complete, some stick around like mercenaries on a retainer as they can remember how to target specific pathogens. These guys are ready to be recalled to the front line at any time with their kill function reactivated. If they were actual human beings, no doubt they'd be fronting TV survival shows.

Test-firing the weapons

The adaptive immune system rarely forgets. This means subsequent exposure to pathogens culminates in a stronger and faster immune response. Thankfully, it also means some infections like measles you typically only get once. Crucially, it is this adaptive immune system that we attempt to hijack when we receive vaccinations.

By exposing your body to components of pathogens in a way that doesn't give you an infection or make you sick, your immune system is provoked into a simulated battle. This leaves it familiar with the face of the enemy and primed for the real war to come.

Although this smart, adaptive system protects us from major infections – and notably death – it has a tendency to overreact. This can result in dozens of autoimmune conditions, from type 1 diabetes to coeliac disease.

There has been an inordinate rise in such health issues over the past few decades, which has been linked to the increased use of antibiotics and a less diverse, more heavily processed diet.

Save yourself

The idea of 'boosting' your immune system is misleading. It sounds good, but an overactive immune system can lead to problems such as allergies or autoimmune diseases like multiple sclerosis. Instead, what you really want to be doing is optimising the existing system. But what can you do that will actually make a difference?

Firstly, a little exposure to the bad stuff can actually be a good thing. Every time you interlace your tongue with another human during a kiss, you also swap somewhere in the realms of 80 million bacteria. Double dipping your Dorito into the communal salsa dip allows the bacterial exchange process to occur, as does standing near someone and speaking to them. This should be reassuring, though you still can't help yourself to my chips.

I won't detail all the benefits of a healthy and balanced diet for your immune system. You've heard it all before and no doubt just want to be left to eat your nibbles in peace. But there's one food group which can make a big difference, and most people in the western world aren't getting enough. Fibre doesn't just promote the microbes in your gut that help to break down food; it also trains your immune system to fight off infections. These gut microbes act as a primary defence barrier against diseases and produce important micronutrients like vitamin K, which supports efficient functioning of the immune system. Oats, wholegrains, baked beans, apples and bananas are full of the stuff so there's no need to break the bank on goji berries and chia seeds to reach your recommended 30g of fibre a day.

In addition, brightly coloured food items like citrus fruits, red cabbage, peppers and berries contain a high number of flavonoids. These are plant-based chemical compounds that can help you fight illness and inflammation.

Backing up your diet with a sensible exercise routine and good sleep health will all benefit your immune system. Finally, you'll need to cut back on the booze. Sorry, but alcohol can suppress your defences and reduce the numbers of good microbes in your gut.

At the end of the day, though, these kinds of lifestyle changes are quite a lot of effort. Surely there must be a shortcut?

Let's consider vitamin C. It's involved in lots of important bodily functions, including the production and activity of white blood cells. As a result, not getting enough of it severely impairs our ability to fight off infections. But – and it's a big but – most people in wealthy countries get all the vitamin C they need from their diet. Even a single kiwi contains more than 100 per cent of the NHS daily recommended intake of the stuff. As our bodies can't store vitamin C, any excess is going to end up being flushed down the loo (just like all that money you spent on the supplements). While there's very little evidence to suggest that taking vitamin C supplements will stop you from getting sick, if you've already got a cold, taking them regularly *can* reduce how long it lasts, even if only by about 8 per cent. In other words, you could shave about ten hours of sniffles off a five-day cold. Think how many tissues you could save.

But before you go popping a whole tube of vitamin C tablets, be aware that it can lead to some serious health problems like diarrhoea, nausea and kidney stones. For this reason, it's recommended you don't have more than 2000mg a day.

Some of these vitamin C supplements have partnered up with another micronutrient. Zinc is a mineral that helps our cellular soldiers bind to and attack infected cells. If taken within the first twenty-four hours of developing cold symptoms, zinc supplements *can* actually make quite a big difference to the length and severity of the infection. A daily dose of zinc has been shown to make recovery from colds three times faster, with 22 per cent less sneezing and half as much coughing. But taking it with vitamin C in one of those fizzy orange tablets isn't going to cut it: zinc supplements are only really effective if they're taken as lozenges which you suck at the back of your throat. The catch is that you have to take quite a lot of zinc to make a difference – around 80mg a day – which is considerably more than you'd find in most supplements (and 10 times your daily recommended intake) What's more, ingesting in excess of 80mg can cause problems, including digestive issues and copper deficiency (which causes anaemia and *reduces* white blood cell counts; exactly the opposite of what you want to be doing).

Vitamin C and zinc have been marketed as cold-crushing cure-alls for decades, but there's also a new kid on the block: vitamin D. This isn't actually a vitamin: it's a hormone that promotes the absorption of calcium in the body. It's also involved in balancing our immune systems, helping our cellular soldiers fight off infections while reducing inflammation and our likelihood of developing autoimmune conditions. Despite this, nearly 1 billion people worldwide aren't getting enough of it. Unlike most vitamins, we only get about 10 per cent of our daily vitamin D requirements from our diets, from oily fish, red meat, eggs and fortified foods like cereals. The biggest source of vitamin D takes the form of sunshine.

Anyone who's ever spent a winter in a country far from the equator will know why this is a problem. During wintertime in the UK, for example, we don't receive enough UV radiation from the sun to produce all the vitamin D our bodies need. As a result, the NHS recommends taking 10μg of vitamin D supplements a day between October and March. This is particularly important if you have darker skin because the pigment melanin prevents what little UV light there is from getting through to where it needs to be.

As with other vitamins, it's also possible to have too much of a good thing – overdosing on vitamin D causes dangerous calcium build-ups in the body, which can weaken bones and damage the kidneys and heart. The good news is that if you stick to under 100μg of the stuff (10 times the recommended daily amount) you're unlikely to have any problems.

Antibiotic apocalypse

One of the greatest achievements in modern medicine must surely be Alexander Fleming's creation of penicillin in the late 1920s and the flurry of antibiotics that followed in the subsequent decades. This a poisoned chalice, however. Undoubtedly, antibiotics are lifesaving when used appropriately, and yet overuse promotes the evolution of superbugs. It can also disturb the natural harmony of your internal ecology and contribute to the evolution of autoimmune issues. So, could it be that this miracle of medicine might be responsible for our downfall? The clock ticks ever closer to the post-antibiotic apocalypse. A world where once again even a simple cut might be lethal. For such a sophisticated modern world, how did we allow ourselves to get here, and what can we do about it?

The answer, to be blunt, originates in ignorance. Little did we know that antibiotics were a precious resource. We handed them out like sweets and unwittingly gave the bacteria a chance to evolve and become resistant. This is because when bacteria are exposed to antibiotics, those with mutations tend to escape such a targeted attack. Potentially these mutant microbes can then reproduce to create a population of super-resistant bacteria. It isn't just humans that can host this resistance movement. We use antibiotics in animal feed and water to prevent outbreaks of livestock disease . . . you can see where this is going. In this alternative post-antibiotic timeline – let's call it a worst-case scenario that might be worth a bet – drug-resistant infections kill 10 million people a year. It's a world in which chemotherapy is unsafe and simple surgeries are too risky to perform. Pneumonia could be unstoppable.

We've had this hate–hate relationship with bacteria for a long time, but actually these ancient creatures have been around far longer than us. With gut health in mind, you could argue that they allow us to function in the way we do today. We enjoy a peaceful symbiosis with them most of the time, but the commercial antibiotics we use are indiscriminate. They may have killed off the bad bacteria but they also destroy many of the other beneficial microbes in your gut's microbiome that help to crowd out more malevolent microbes like *Salmonella*, *Campylobacter* and *Clostridum difficile*.

Thankfully, we have some solutions to the looming antibiotic crisis. Advances in science means we can focus on proofing them against resistance, and yet there is also hope from the natural world. One potential saviour is a type of virus called bacteriophage. These ancient creatures are the most abundant organism in the world. They're harmless to humans and exist to invade other viruses, reproduce and effectively destroy them. Fungi is another hopeful candidate in the fight against antibiotics as we know some produce chemicals that kill bacteria. A great deal of hope is resting on these developments, because without them we might well be doomed.

I am not suggesting that we stop using antibiotics altogether. We just need to get smarter about when and how we use them. For example, antibiotics are meant to treat bacterial diseases. They are useless against viral diseases like colds and flu, and yet in parts of the world where antibiotics are available off the shelf it's considered the first line of defence. For now, the war rages on. It's an arms race between bacteria and antibiotics that continues to gather speed. How it plays out, well . . . we can only hope there's a happy ending.

The saboteur

What happens when the immune system goes rogue? Exactly how does it feel when the guards attack the body they're meant to defend? This is the essence of autoimmune disease and it happens more frequently than many recognise.

We're talking about a fine example of a task failed successfully. Autoimmune disease is a bit like letting loose a bunch of sugar-crazy toddlers on cleaning the dishes. They'll throw themselves into the task, only to smash everything. When the smart targeting system of immunity fails in a healthy host, it mounts an inflammatory response. The result is damage caused to healthy tissue. A dramatic example of this are autoimmune conditions like lupus or inflammatory bowel diseases like Crohn's or ulcerative colitis. In going rogue, the immune system recognises normal body cells as foreign and mounts an attack against them. It's an anti-sickness system that has become the cause of the sickness itself.

From a medical perspective, autoimmune diseases are frustrating to deal with. Why? Because there is no clear tumour to cut out, no bacteria to kill with antibiotics and no virus to quell with antibodies. The villain is you. It's an extreme example of friendly fire gone wrong. When your body attacks itself (you), often the only solution is to suppress the entire immune system. Naturally, this leaves you at higher risk of other infections. Sometimes the treatment is as bad as the disease.

As a final cruelty in this strange and often remorseless self-sabotage, autoimmune conditions disproportionally affect more women than men. What's more, due to the chronicity of the symptoms, depression and other mental health issues often accompanies them. I wish I could tell you there was some evolutionary trade-off which meant that autoimmune disease has some benefit but alas, no. It is an error in the immune system; a malfunction that we can only hope will become a thing of the past as medicine evolves.

Peanuts on the plane

For a strong, resilient defence set-up, your immune system can be quite the princess if it bumps into something harmless like pollen or gluten and irrationally decides to take a dislike to it.

Generally, allergies may not be as life-altering as some autoimmune diseases. Even so, they do share a commonality. In both cases, your immune system malfunctions and loses the plot. From a common-sense perspective as much as a medical one, allergies are insane. Your body triggers such an aggressive immune response to a harmless substance that it could kill you. Overreaction? You could say that.

Nowadays it seems as if everyone is allergic to something. Unfortunately, not all allergies are created equally. You might have an innocuous intolerance to a particular food that causes a tingle in the mouth or an itchy tongue, or full-blown, life-threatening anaphylaxis in the case of severe nut allergies.

Are we too clean?

During the last century, we came to the realisation that not all microbes are bad. The majority are harmless; in fact, many can be beneficial. This notion gave rise to the 'hygiene hypothesis' that postulates that our squeaky clean environments, in which we wall off children and ourselves from all manner of microbial agents, may have negative consequences to the immune system.

Now, this doesn't quite tell the whole story. The idea we need to be less hygienic is inherently wrong. Relaxing hygiene standards would in fact be a backwards step. For one thing, it would diminish the playground of hard knocks where your immune system learns to toughen up. But as a child your developing immune system takes cues from all the minor encounters in your life., from playing in the dirt or sleeping over at a friend's house to eating food that has been dropped on your kitchen floor. In a society with diminishing chances of these encounters, your primed but relatively untested immune system could well become trigger-happy. The solution is to just be sensible. Go out. Meet people. Enjoy life. Just wash your hands when appropriate, avoid guzzling antibiotics at the slightest sniffle and try not to sleep in dog shit.

Save yourself

On a cellular level, there might not be much you can do to influence your immune system's lifelong war campaign. Where you can enlist in the good fight, however, is by bolstering your first lines of defence.

Your body is filled with various orifices, holes, cracks and crevices. Pathogens like viruses and bacteria take advantage of darkness, moisture and your sticky surfaces to cause chaos over a wider arena. Some of these agents even hijack the mucosal linings of your nose, throat, lungs – and even the intestines – to trigger bouts of coughing, sneezing and diarrhoea. In doing so, they replicate themselves and then dispatch into the wider world to infect your fellow humans.

You can avoid being complicit in these heinous acts by ensuring you cover your face holes when coughing or sneezing. If you're feeling under the weather, it wouldn't be a bad idea to revive that lockdown look by wearing a mask when out and about.

Your body is also lined with secret passages that connect all sorts of plumbing apparatuses. For example, there's the nasolacrimal duct which runs from the lacrimal punctum at the corners of your eyelids down to your nose. This pipe allows tears to drain which is why you sometimes get a runny nose when you cry. Dangerously, this same duct also has a secret connection to the sinuses as well as the middle ear via the eustachian tube. As you love to touch your face and eyeballs for some odd reason, a virus or pathogenic microbe from your finger could swiftly flit to your eyeball, and from there the duct will deliver it deep into your body. The most effective solution is to wash your hands on a regular basis, and basically stop touching your face. By curtailing what is no doubt the habit of a lifetime, you could even be saving yourself from an early grave.

The case against cancer

If you've managed to duck and dodge all manner of infectious beasts that stalk mankind, there is a threat of one cruel monster that lingers over all humans.

Cancer rates have steadily climbed in humans because, well, we've got good at not being killed by other things. This means the longer we stay alive the greater the chance your immune system fails to kill a rogue cell is the biological equivalent of leaving the oven on.

You could argue cancer is the worst design flaw of all. It is possible to reduce the risk of cancer, screen for it, treat, cut out, irradiate and poison it, but with current science it's still impossible to eliminate the risk entirely. Why? Because it exists where cells exist and wherever cell replication occurs.

Another reason there is no universal 'cure' for cancer is because of the frequently misunderstood nature of what it is. Cancer is an umbrella term that encompasses hundreds of wildly different pathologies. It isn't one entity, it's a disease process. Every cancer – even within the same organ type such as the breast or bladder – is markedly different in terms of its genetic make-up. Cancer is as unique as the DNA within you.

Similar to autoimmune disease, cancer occurs when your own cells turn rogue. It means they cease obeying the laws that govern them, and refuse to stop growing when instructed. Instead, like unrest without purpose, they multiply into a dangerous mob. Occasionally, if left unchecked, cancer can jump on various internal transport systems and scam itself a trip to other parts of your body. The spread of cancer is known as metastasis. It's a process that can progressively cripple the body due to the increased metabolic demand of cancer cells and gradual loss of function of the various systems it hijacks.

Cancer is hard to treat because it's not about expelling an invader but eradicating an insurrection from within. Treatment is effectively an attack on yourself. In removing a bowel cancer, for example, us surgeons also have to chop out a margin of normal healthy tissue. Then there's chemotherapy, which blitzes healthy cells too.

The immune system can't be scapegoated for missing early cancers all the time. After all, almost every cell in the body experiences random genetic mutations and frequently these are a result of toxins from your environment. During my time at medical school, when revising for the written component of my finals, I was faced with this question: 'A 75-year-old man who used to work in a factory working with aniline dyes has been complaining of weight loss, blood in the urine, and abdominal pain. What is the most likely diagnosis?' There was a list of answers but reflexively I had been trained to recognise that bladder cancer is often caused by work-related toxins.

Save yourself

Cancer strikes fear into all our hearts, and with good reason. In stark contrast to many things that can kill us, it often rears its mutated head without any warning signs. While there is very little you can do to prevent cancer, it is possible to mitigate some risk factors associated with lifestyle. Several might seem obvious, but the causal link is so strong that spelling them out might save your life.

Smoking is perhaps one of the biggest villains in the line-up. Even one cigarette can damage your DNA, which is the trigger for cancer. Smoking can cause cancers of essentially every tissue and organ in your body, from pancreas to liver to ovary and even some forms of leukaemia. E-cigarettes haven't been on the block as long as tobacco, so it's difficult to make firm conclusions about the association with cancer risk. What we do know is that vapours from certain e-cigarettes can contain carcinogens, which is the name for any cancer-causing agent.

Alcohol consumption is also associated with cancer, while cutting down your intake or quitting altogether has wider benefits for your health. A balanced, high-fibre diet and regular exercise is also proven to help bolster your body's defences, as are good sleeping habits. A massive respect for the power of the sun will also reduce your risk of developing skin cancer (melanomas), which means applying sunscreen even on days with thin cloud cover. As nobody is immune from cancer, your body will thank you for putting it through regular screenings by a health professional. Your GP can advise on an appropriate programme.

To finish your tour of duty through the immune system, let's be both clear and reasonable here. Despite the shortcomings, it's still a pretty good defensive shield. If it was totally shoddy at its job we would have long succumbed to the inordinate number of murderous microbes that linger around you like vultures. In reality it wins trillions of battles for you every day of your life. In fact, your immune system is so well adapted it pretty much comes with a guarantee to pick up on 99.9 per cent of all attacks. Don't celebrate too early, however, because that leaves a daily count of about ten million that go undetected.

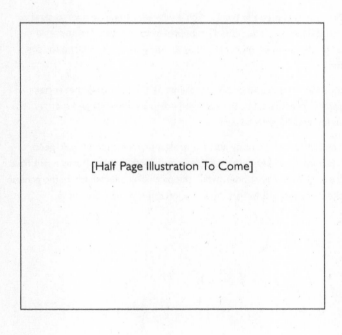

[Half Page Illustration To Come]

Health Hack

Nobody is immune to pain, which is why we often reach for analgaesic medication like paracetamol or ibuprofen to reduce or relieve mild or moderate discomfort caused by anything from a headache to sore muscles.

It can be tempting to ignore the claims on the packaging that certain painkillers act fast, but this is a tightly regulated market and such statements have to be legit.

The fact is that the body absorbs analgaesic medication in salt, gel or liquid form quicker than the tablet variety. While these forms might have the edge in terms of how swiftly the painkilling effects kick in, the generic cheaper ones will still get the same job done in their own time.

14. This Is the End

DIGGING UP THE FACTS
ABOUT DEATH

IT WAS MY SECOND GRAVEYARD SHIFT in a row, or maybe my third. Even though I'd only recently qualified as a doctor, I still felt like I was just dressing up in scrubs with a stethoscope around my neck. My beeper had just gone off, inviting me to pick up a request to certify a patient's death. This is something I had observed but never performed myself. In that moment, I felt a weight of responsibility I had never experienced before. Solemnly, but with a sense of purpose, I walked down the dark corridors of the ward and located the side room of the recently deceased patient: an elderly woman who had died of pneumonia.

There was a stillness in the room I hadn't felt before. The body was at the heart of that stillness, expressionless and draped in a hospital gown. Although I'd seen death before, her open eyes seemingly met my gaze when I hovered over her.

I reminded myself of the steps required to certify a patient's death. First, I touched a piece of tissue paper on to the patient's cornea, the outermost part of the eye, to elicit a sudden blinking (known as the corneal reflex). It was absent. Next, I shone a pen-torch into her eyes. The pupils were motionless and fixed instead of shrinking and dilating like they would in response to light and darkness respectively. Then I squeezed the trapezius muscle, covering the shoulder, and also applied pressure to the sternum.

There was no response from either test.

Next it was time to listen to the chest through my stethoscope. I was twenty-four years old. Since entering medicine, I'd encountered various forms of death: the brutal failed resuscitation efforts of a 94-year-old woman, the on-table cardiac arrest of a patient during surgery, the anonymous, formaldehyde-soaked bodies in the dissection lab. This was different. Just half an hour before, my patient was still breathing. She passed away without commotion, her body succumbing to an unrelenting chest infection.

My stethoscope picked up noises. It startled me briefly. Then I registered that it was caused by interference from my hand moving. When I anchored it firmly, I heard nothing but unsettling silence. I was required to listen for four minutes. In that time, my mind filled with thoughts about this woman's life: her childhood, loved ones and final thoughts as she left this world. I didn't know her, or even encounter her in life, and yet I felt a profound responsibility towards her in that moment. Once I confirmed the death, I lifted the sheets to cover her body, like a parent tucking in their child, and then retreated from the room. Before returning to the hustle, bustle and beeps of a busy ward, I closed the door as if not to wake her.

Death isn't always a defeat. Sometimes, it is a natural conclusion resulting from medicine's limitations and the inevitable progression of disease or age. Although I'd completed this one job, and faced a mountain of others before my shift was complete, I acknowledged that her passing was more than a tick-box. It was, I realised, an encounter with an elemental force that I continue to meet in the course of my career, and which one day will come for me.

The price of a long life

Once upon a time, humans were bestowed around three decades of life on earth before relinquishing their mortal coils and expiring. Over the last two hundred years or so, however, us meat machines have extended our use-by dates significantly. Today, at the age of thirty, you are no longer reaching the end of your life like your predecessors. Instead, you are probably just at the beginning stages of 'adulting'.

Human bodies have been through the rigmarole of various disease and self-destruction, from typhoid to tobacco addiction, but still stand proudly. Since the advent of farming and agriculture, and also settling closer to animals, we effectively surrounded ourselves with new illnesses, which was the first of many mistakes. Then, in gravitating towards dense urban clusters riddled with poor sanitation, we created breeding grounds for pestilence. In the fourteenth century, the Black Death wiped out between 30 and 60 per cent of the European population. We fought back through proper hygiene measures, vaccines and later antibiotics but our increased life expectancy has come at a price. Yes, we can live for long enough to lecture younger generations about how it was better in our day, but in doing so we invite cancers, heart disease and strokes into our elderly lives.

Let there be ... life?

Doctors have always been intrigued by the boundaries between life and death. In 1774, such interest led to the foundation of the Royal Humane Society in London. Known at the time as the Society for the Recovery of Persons Apparently Drowned, their aim was to develop and disseminate information on how to perform lifesaving first aid with the aim of bringing people back from death's door.

At the time, mouth-to-mouth resuscitation was considered a vulgar practice. This was in sharp contrast to the use of tobacco enemas, in which tobacco smoke was literally pumped up the dying person's anus with a set of bellows and considered to be completely acceptable. There are a small number of reports that this procedure actually worked. From a modern medical perspective, it's more likely that the patients were startled back to life by having hot air pumped up their arse. If true, I imagine a percentage must have promptly died of indignity.

Happily, the Royal Humane Society also encouraged more conventional treatments, namely the use of electricity to shock the victims back to consciousness. A report from the society in 1794 described how, after falling out of a second-story window, a child called Sophia Greenhill was brought back from the brink by the application of electricity to her chest

Believe it or not, the use of electricity in medicine dates back to antiquity: Ancient Roman physicians used the electric shocks from black torpedo fish to treat everything from headaches to gout to a prolapsed anus. It wasn't until the eighteenth century, however, that we were really able to harness the power of electricity for ourselves.

An Italian physician called Luigi Galvani was the first of many to demonstrate electricity's ability to stimulate movement in dead bodies. We're talking frogs here, not people (yet). He showed how live wires attached to the nerves and muscles of deceased amphibians would cause their lifeless limbs to twitch vigorously. His nephew, Giovanni Aldini, took these death-defying demonstrations one step further. It begins on a freezing morning in 1803, when the murderer, George Forster, was hung from the gallows at London's Newgate prison. Seconds after drawing his last breath, Forster's limp body was rushed off to the Royal College of Surgeons in London, where he was laid out on a long stone slab in the middle of the operating theatre. Pacing beside it was Aldini. In his hands he clasped two metal wires attached to a tall column of metal plates, which was the closest thing they had to the pocket-sized lithium batteries we use today. As the chattering among his nervous onlookers died down, Aldini attached the two wires to the dead man's temples and fired up his metal contraption.

Immediately, Forster's face contorted violently and his left eye snapped open. The crowd gasped and jumped back in their seats. But Aldini simply smiled and calmly let go of the wires. The body fell still. Next he moved one of the wires to the dead man's ear while sticking the other one up his anus (apparently this was totally cool, but mouth-to-mouth resuscitation still much too fruity). Bringing the wire ends to his shining metal tower he completed the circuit once more. This time, the corpse's legs began to kick, his back arched and his clenched right fist punched vigorously into the air. Many of his onlookers felt they had witnessed a miracle, even though Aldini had not been able to restart the corpse's heart. Indeed, once he removed the wires the body became lifeless once more.

News of this dramatic demonstration travelled across Europe, and it's likely that a young Mary Shelley got wind of Aldini's electrifying endeavours. Thirteen years later she went on to write her world-famous novel, *Frankenstein*.

This whole 'spark of life' thing made for some impressive demonstrations and was responsible for one of the most seminal pieces of literature of the nineteenth century. But how legit is the science behind all this? Well, believe it or not, it's actually a lot more reasonable than you might think. The work of Galvani and his ambitious nephew eventually opened the door on research into the essential role of electricity in all living things. The fact is it powers your every movement and thought, your heartbeat and even consciousness itself. In some people, particularly after surgery or a heart attack, these signals can become out of sync. This can cause the heart to beat too fast or too slow, or without any clear rhythm at all. In these cases, the patient might be fitted with an artificial pacemaker, a small device that is implanted in the patient's chest and sends electrical signals to the heart to tell it when to beat normally. In many ways Galvani was quite the visionary, for we now use defibrillators to resuscitate people who are clinically dead. In many ways, electricity is the essence of life. Without it, there is darkness.

Preparing for death

Many of us live our lives like we are immortal. Anti-ageing has become a popular commercial pursuit and there's no doubt today we squeeze out every last drop of life that our bodied can support. As a result, because death can seem such a long way away, our language surrounding the topic has become abstract and sanitised.

I realise my profession might seem peculiar. I am involved in the process of prolonging life, but death can sometimes have the upper hand. Just like an office water cooler, corpses are a familiar feature of my workplace. We don't congregate around them at break times to gossip or anything, but if I encounter death on a shift it doesn't shock me to the core like it did that first time.

While I have a deep, personal and long-standing insight into death, I am aware that most people haven't ever seen a dead body. In my mind, it makes coming face to face with death somewhat challenging, whether you're close to the end yourself or connected to other with limited time left. We've even created an entire lexicon around euphemising it. We don't die or expire. We pass away, rest in peace or cross the rainbow bridge, as if to suggest there's something awaiting us on the other side. We use such terms as emollients to soothe and manage the process of death, and yet sometimes that just conspires to reinforce the taboo around it.

It's important to face the inescapable truth that your body at some point must be broken down and recycled. At the end of life, the great green bin awaits us all. Ultimately, if we're going to face the topic of mortality with freedom then we cannot squirm away from it. We can still treat it with humour as much as respect. We just have to face the facts in order to come to terms with it.

Avoiding the reality about death can be harmful. Just look what happens when we try to ban stuff we don't like, such as alcohol in prohibition America, cannabis or Frankie Goes to Hollywood. There will still be a demand for death because biology dictates that our bodies have a shelf life. We can just choose whether or not to embrace it with honesty and ultimately make peace with the inevitable — whenever that may be.

Save yourself

Whether you're fit and healthy or living with a terminal illness, learning to talk about death can be curiously comforting. By making the unspoken an everyday subject, death loses the air of fear and uncertainty that can haunt us all. In fact, embracing the subject can bring peace of mind, from crucial conversations between loved ones, knowing time is running out, to practical decision-making in a bid to regain control of your future final chapter (such as making a will or choosing whether to be resuscitated in the event of an otherwise terminal episode).

When are you actually dead?

Seeing that you're asking a medical practitioner, I will argue there are two different kinds of death: clinical and biological.

Clinical death is when you stop breathing and your blood stops flowing. So, you're pretty dead, but in some cases this kind of death is still reversible. Take Audrey Schoeman, a British woman who developed severe hypothermia while hiking in a snowstorm in the Spanish Pyrenees mountains. She was clinically dead for six hours before she eventually regained consciousness. Then there was Janina Kolkiewicz, a 91-year-old Polish woman, who spent eleven hours in cold storage at a morgue before waking up to complain that she was cold and wanted pancakes.

In fact, enough people have spontaneously regained heart function after being clinical dead that the phenomenon has earned its own name: Lazarus syndrome. Incredibly, 35 per cent of people with this condition manage to return to a normal, healthy life afterwards.

Setting aside the terror associated with that concept, how do we know when someone is properly *dead* dead? Here, we turn our attention to the second kind of death: biological death. This happens when a patient has no remaining brain activity. Once you are brain dead, there's no coming back.

It sounds cut and dried, and yet brain-dead patients can continue to function, albeit not very effectively, in the absence of brain activity. Indeed, the heart of a brain-dead patient can continue to beat for hours, or even days, after brain activity stops. One pregnant woman was kept on life support for 117 days after her brain activity had stopped so that her unborn foetus could continue to develop inside of her. After a good deal of medical handholding, her healthy baby girl was delivered via C-section on day eleven. From tragedy came life.

Conversely, brain activity can also continue for some time after the heart has stopped beating. Studying this activity could give us an idea of what really goes on in someone's head after they've drawn their last breath. The first evidence of post-mortem brain activity was discovered accidentally after an 87-year-old man suffered a heart attack while undergoing a continuous electroencephalography scan (used to monitor brain waves). His EEG revealed ongoing activity recorded on the scan even after the point at which the man's heart stopped beating. Even more interesting is the fact that these types of brain waves are the same as those we have when we are dreaming and during memory retrieval. So, it's very possible that in his last few moments before the monitor showed no further activity, the man literally saw his life flashing before his eyes.

As much as we'd like to draw a nice, clear line between life and death, it's just not that straightforward. Death is not a singular event. It's a gradual process of shutting down that can go on for hours, even days.

What happens after death?

That old chestnut. Well, on a purely physical level, and without wandering into the realms of philosophy or science fiction, your body literally feasts on itself. The ever willing and helpful bacteria and enzymes that were once so useful turn on you and begin to digest you from the inside out. It's a morbid thought, but it has to be better than being alive when they set about consuming you. So, how are these miniature carnivores kept in check? For this, you can thank one of life's essentials . . . blood.

Your body is kept somewhat happy throughout life by the fact that blood transports oxygen and nutrients to your cells and smuggles away waste products. When you die, blood no longer pumps around. Subsequently the cells are deprived of nutrition and oxygen, accumulate waste and undergo a precipitous drop in pH value. We're talking about a measure of alkalinity and acidity here, and in this case it's simpler to think of it in terms of power fizzing through an electrified fence. This serves to contain the wild monsters within the cells, which take the form of enzymes. Once the pH drops, the cell membranes become useless. As a result, the monsters escape.

Once this membrane is breached upon your death, these enzymes ransack the cell and begin the digestive process known as autolysis. This process is particularly swift and violent in organs rich in enzymes such as the pancreas, stomach and liver, but ultimately no cell in the body escapes such a devouring. The living can even witness this process in action. Rigor mortis is one the most unsettling manifestations of death, in which the changing chemical structure within the muscles of a corpse causes them to stiffen. The process can last for up to twelve hours, and can be a useful tool for pathologists in determining the time of death. Eventually, the muscles relax, but essentially this is down to the fact that the enzymes have begun to consume their structure. We're talking about a stage of decomposition here. It also gets worse.

Next comes the deluge of bacteria, and there's a lot of them. In fact, your body has more bacterial cells than human cells. When you're alive, your immune system keeps these prisoners under control. When these guards are relieved from duty upon your death, the convicts run wild. Unopposed, they begin the feast that the enzymes have prepared in advance. This is putrefaction. In this process, the bacteria feast on your tissues and release pungent gaseous emissions like methane. This can cause an unsightly bloating of your body. At this point, it wouldn't take a medical expert to determine that you really are dead.

Donating your body to science

If you really have breathed your last, and there's no coming back from it, then I am sorry about your death. But fear not, if you'd prefer not to decompose, or go up in flames at the crematorium, then you could donate your body to medical science. We'll take good care of you.

We know there is a great deal of grief, trauma and loss surrounding death. It's part of what makes us human. At the same time, we are still advancing as a species, and in order to continue the dead can still teach us a great deal. Donated bodies allow medical students, trainee surgeons and even established ones to practise and gain expertise on procedures as simple as learning anatomy to complex surgeries like bowel cancer operations.

Save others

Technically speaking, as a dead person you're beyond help at this point. Before you go, however, if the prospect of donating your body to science on death appeals then talk to your GP about registering. While it might not be for everyone, I can safely say that without cadavers to learn from, thanks to kind-hearted souls over the years I would not be a doctor today, let alone a surgeon.

On a final note, while everything I've told you thus far is steeped in science, medicine and personal hospital experience, the truth is everything could turn out to be utterly wrong. In years from now, medical advances could make a mockery of this book. We still have many more mysteries to uncover about the human body and problems to solve surrounding its inbuilt lethality. If you consider how much of human existence revolves around rest, repair, extended periods of maintenance and wiping your arse, you can see this actually makes the good moments even better.

It's also worth remembering what a miracle you are. For a heap of alien space dust flung into the reaches of infinite space, which settled on a warm rock, led to single-celled life on planet earth and then painstakingly, mistake after mistake, evolved to come up with you, against all odds you've come a long way. So, despite the fact that you're playing a small part in a grand work in progress called the human race, and living with odd body quirks, vestigial traits and random mutations, I urge you to go out and enjoy your time on earth. After all, you could be an ant that unwittingly brings poisoned food back to its anthill and ends up killing the entire colony and the queen. In this view, life is not that bad after all.

NOTES

4 Pages To Come

Notes

Notes

Notes

ACKNOWLEDGEMENTS

2 Pages To Come

Acknowledgements

PICTURE CREDITS

To Come

INDEX

Index

Index

Index